UNSHAKABLE

Unlocking Your Blueprint to Living Well Despite Limitations

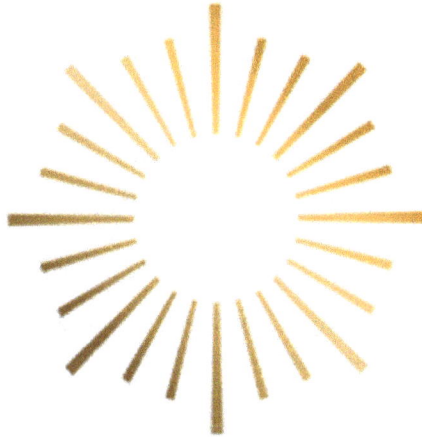

SONYA MCDONALD

Board Certified Transformational Life Coach, RN, BSN, BCC

ISBN: 978-1-968061-45-6

A Note To The Reader

My hope is that this book becomes more than just words on a page—it becomes your turning point. A lifeline. A blueprint. What you're holding is not just my story—it's the system I used to heal, rise, and reclaim my energy and life. Inside these pages is **The Energy Intelligence Method™**—my 9-pillar blueprint that helped me go from stuck and inflamed to free and unshakable.

If you're tired of being tired, if you feel like you're holding it all together for everyone but silently breaking inside, I want you to know this: you are not broken. You are not behind. You are not too late. There is a way forward—and you are holding it in your hands.

If someone you love is silently struggling, burned out, or buried under the weight of invisible battles, share this with them. Together, let's make sure no woman is left in the dark about her worth, her healing, or her power.

This journey only works if we show up honestly and fully. That's what I promise to do in these pages. I'm not here to impress you. I'm here to walk with you. My prayer is that you won't just read this book—you'll live it. That it will become the blueprint you return to every time life tries to shake you.

When I imagine a world where women stop defining themselves by their pain, diagnoses, or limitations, I see a movement. A ripple of resilience, healing, and truth that starts with one light being ignited at a time. If this book lights something up in you, don't keep it to yourself. Share it. Post it. Pass it on. Someone out there is praying for the hope you now hold.

We are not meant to do this alone. I may be the author, but **you** are the reason this book matters. I am so grateful for your courage to rise. Whether this is your rock bottom or your comeback season, I want you to know—your healing is possible. Your energy is reclaimable. And your story isn't over.

If something in these pages speaks to your soul, I'd love for you to share it on social media using the hashtags #UnshakableBook or #IgniteYourLight. Tag me so I can cheer you on. You never know who you'll inspire to stop hiding and start healing.

You can connect with me at SonyaMcDonald.com, where you can book a free Energy Health Assessment and take your first step toward a more energized, peaceful, and aligned life. Follow me on social media for daily encouragement, and scan the QR code below to connect instantly.

Food, movement, mindset, and faith are our most powerful forms of medicine. They are not just habits—they are healing fuel. When you combine them with purpose, transformation becomes inevitable. I'm here to be your guide to help you get there.

Let's elevate your energy, double your peace, and learn to move through life with less stress and more authentic living, where you can live well despite any challenge. This is your time to rise into a life that's vibrant, empowered, and truly unshakable.

Ignite your light. Transform your life. Live an unshakable life.

Please note: This book is not intended to replace therapy or medical treatment. It is a reflection of lived experience, healing tools, and transformational truth to support your journey.

Scan QR Code

Sonya McDonald

Introduction

There's a moment in life where everything shifts.

A moment where you realize you can't keep living the same way, where you're tired of just surviving and ready to truly live. For me, that moment came when I was lying in a hospital bed, my body exhausted, my mind overwhelmed, my spirit broken.

I had spent years fighting, pushing, trying to "fix" my health, but no matter what I did, I felt like I was slipping further away from the life I wanted. And in that moment of complete surrender, I made a decision that changed everything.

I decided that I would no longer let my limitations define me.

I decided that I would reclaim my power, no matter what.

I decided that I would become Unshakable.

My life as a Registered Nurse gave me a deep understanding of the human body and the layers of illness. Yet, even with my medical knowledge, I found myself helpless against the relentless assault of chronic pain.

My own personal experience with Rheumatoid Arthritis and Fibromyalgia provided an intimate understanding of the challenges faced by those living with chronic invisible illness.

And now?

I'm here to show you how to do the same.

What This Book Is Really About

This book isn't just about my journey.

It's about yours.

It's for the woman who feels stuck in survival mode, who knows she's meant for more but doesn't know how to get there, who has let fear, self-doubt, or past struggles keep her small. Because I know what it's like to feel like life is happening to you instead of you creating it.

Unshakable isn't only a clinical account; it's a deeply personal narrative, an exploration of physical healing, as well as emotional and spiritual transformation. And while this book speaks directly to women, it is also for anyone who loves, supports, or walks alongside them.

Whether you're a father, brother, partner, son, friend, or simply someone seeking a deeper understanding and transformation of your own, this book offers insights and reflections that speak to all, regardless of gender, because healing, growth, and purpose are human experiences we all deserve to claim.

I know what it's like to let illness, exhaustion, or fear steal your joy. To wonder if you'll ever feel strong, energized, or at peace again.

And I also know what it takes to break free.

You Were Made for More

The biggest lie we tell ourselves is that we must accept our limitations as permanent. That we are powerless to change our reality. That healing, whether physical, emotional, or spiritual, is out of reach.

But I'm here to tell you: You are stronger than you've been led to believe. You are capable of transforming your life. You were made for more than just surviving; you were made to thrive.

This book isn't here to inspire you for a moment and then fade away. It's here to give you the blueprint to reclaim your life.

Through this transformational memoir, I aim to share my journey, highlighting not only the practical strategies that helped me regain control of my health, like dietary changes, increased physical activity, mindful listening to my body, and an unshakable shift in mindset, but also the emotional roller coaster of hope, despair, and ultimately, triumph.

What You'll Learn in These Pages

In Unshakable, I'm going to walk you through the exact steps that took me from feeling completely broken, lost, and stuck to living fully, fearlessly, and with unshakable strength.

Each chapter offers practical tools and techniques, gathered from both my medical background and personal experience, designed to empower readers to create their own blueprints for thriving, moving beyond mere survival to a life filled with vitality, purpose, and joy.

Together, we'll explore:

- The truth about resilience and why setbacks don't define you.
- How trauma and stress impact your body, and how to release them.
- Daily habits that will restore your energy and peace.
- How to shift your mindset and take control of your healing.
- Why you must protect your energy and set boundaries.

- How to step into your purpose and never look back.

This isn't about "thinking positively" and hoping for the best. This is about rewriting the rules for your life and becoming unstoppable.

This isn't just a memoir; it's a companion, a guide, a source of inspiration and empowerment to help you navigate your own unique path toward a life of vibrant health and fulfilling purpose.

The One Promise I Need You to Make

Before we begin, I need you to make me a promise.

Promise me that you will finish this book.

Promise me that you will show up for yourself, even when it's hard.

Promise me that you won't let fear stop you from stepping into your power.

Because if you're willing to do that, your life will never be the same again.

I didn't write this book to just tell you my story.

I wrote it to help you step into your own transformation.

Remember, healing is not a destination, but a journey, and I'm here to guide you every step of the way.

So, are you ready?

Because your unshakable journey starts now.

Dedication & Acknowledgments

To God—my anchor, my strength, and my light. Thank you for never leaving my side, even when I felt lost in the dark. It was in my deepest surrender that I discovered my truest power. Every word of this book, every step of this journey, is because of Your grace.

There are no words to fully express my gratitude for the people who have stood by me, believed in me, and lifted me through every chapter of my life, especially during the hardest ones. This book is dedicated to my family, my unwavering rock through the storm. Your love, patience, and unconditional support were my lifeline during the darkest days. This journey wouldn't have been possible without your belief in me, even when I had lost faith in myself.

To my beautiful daughters, Sierra and Mia: You are my heart, my light, and my biggest inspiration. You are my why. Your bright smiles remind me of the beauty life holds. Even amidst the pain, you are my inspiration. Every step I take, every word I write, every stage I stand on, I do it for you. I love you both with all my being, to infinity and beyond. You are my reason, and I hope this book reminds you that you, too, are Unshakable.

To my husband, Tyler: Thank you for all your unconditional love, support, and belief in me. You have loved me through my weakest moments and celebrated me in my strongest. I couldn't do this journey without you. I love you beyond measure. I am very grateful to you and for all that you do to make this dream happen for me.

To my Mom and Dad: Your love and guidance laid the foundation for my resilience. Thank you for instilling in me the strength to face any challenge. Thank you for teaching me about faith and the power of never giving up. Your love has shaped me in ways I will always carry with me forever. I love you both so much.

To my brother, Ken, and sister, Jen, thank you for loving me through the storms and cheering for me in the light. Your belief in me helped make this dream take flight. You both mean more to me than words can say. I love you both beyond words.

To Lulu, my sweet miracle dog—you were with me in the quiet moments, the tears, and the breakthroughs. Your presence reminded me that I was never alone. Thank you for loving me through it all.

To Hope Isenberg, you have been by my side on this wild ride of life since our nursing job together over 27 years ago, when we met as nurses and became lifelong best friends! You are always loving, encouraging, and supporting me through every chapter of my life. I'm endlessly grateful for your constant presence and heart. I love you so much.

To Jennifer Jaskal, you have been there through it all, the highs and lows, and every sacred moment in between. I am so grateful to you and that God had us cross paths. He knew exactly what he was doing. You held my hand as I poured my heart into these pages and stood beside me on adventures that helped me make this book a reality. Your unwavering belief in God and me has been a guiding light. I'm beyond blessed to have you in my life and as my best friend. I love you to infinity and beyond.

To Stevi Quick, you may not be physically here, but I still feel you in all I do. I hear you pushing me to keep going, just like you always did. You were a warrior all the way, and your strength still carries me.

To Paul Herber, thank you for your support through it all. Even in pain, we found ways to express and create, sharing what was in our hearts for the world to see. I know Stevi is so proud of all we are doing. Your talent in art continues to inspire, and I am grateful we became friends.

To Angela Green, words can't express how thankful I am to have met you last year. Your belief in me has meant the world. I am so grateful for your support and so happy to have you in my life.

To Shelly Cameron, my joy bringer. You have been a light in my life, always knowing how to lift my spirit, make me laugh, and help me destress when I need it most. Your friendship is a gift from God that I will always cherish. I love you and am forever grateful for you!

To Jillian Arena, words can't even begin to express my gratitude for you, our friendship, and your belief in me! The way we met was pure synchronicity at our beautiful Stevi's celebration of life. I can't begin to tell you how blessed I am to have met you there. You are a light in my life and have helped me so much with your encouragement and just being a genuine friend. I am so thankful for you building my beautiful website and helping me with all the tech along the way. I love you so much!

To Denise Woodson, you have walked this entire journey with me, and your belief in me has meant the world. I love you and I am so grateful for our friendship. You have been a blessing in my life. Here is to all we have overcome–and all that's still ahead.

To Laurie Hamill, you have been the steadfast best friend that I can always count on. Even when life gets busy and the months pass by, we pick up right where we left off, like no time has passed. Your love, loyalty, and quiet strength mean the world to me. I am so grateful for your presence in my life, always. I love you.

To Suzi Dunn, my lifelong friend. I am so thankful for you and our friendship and all our fun adventures, and for more to come. I love you so much.

To Becky Bois, your friendship and being there for me through all of this have been golden and priceless. I am so grateful and thankful to you. I love you so very much.

To Catherine Cherny - I treasure our friendship and thank you for always looking out for me, and for believing in me when I needed it most. Your encouragement through this entire process has meant everything to me. I love and appreciate you so much.

To Alla Friedman and Krisztina Ergas, you two have been such a constant light in my life. Through every high and low, you have shown up with hope, love, and laughter. You have given me a safe place to land, to grow, and to rise again. We truly are the three musketeers - forever lifting each other up, no matter what. I love you both so much.

To all these incredible besties of mine, thank you for loving me through every season, never judging, never walking away, and always showing up with open arms. You have been my anchors, my cheerleaders, and my safe place. I love you more than words can ever say.

To Dr. Kat Maslowe, thank you for being such a blessing in my life. Your encouragement, support, and unwavering belief in me have been truly priceless. You created a safe space where I could be fully myself, and in that space, I found the strength to grow into the woman I was always meant to be. I am so blessed and beyond grateful for you and for always believing in me.

To Hanna Olivas at She Rises Studios, you are a true blessing in my life. Your belief in me and the opportunity you gave me through She Rises

Studios turned my dream into a reality. From the moment I joined, you poured into me, lifted me, and helped me find my voice. Sharing my story on your platform at Empower Her Content Day in Las Vegas was a moment I will never forget. Because of you, I had the courage to rise and write this book and share my message with the world! I am grateful for our friendship, sisterhood, and mentorship. I love you so much!

To Adriana Carlos, my editor, Jhan Ellyza Dimatera, Catherine Cruz, Berna de Jesus, and the entire She Rises Publishing team, thank you for helping me make this book possible. Your dedication, support, and guidance brought my vision to life. I'm grateful beyond words for each of you. Your insightful suggestions and meticulous attention to detail significantly enhanced the clarity and impact of this book.

To all of the She Rises Studios Community, I want to thank each and every single one of you for sharing your hearts, voices, stories, and the impact you have had on my life by being in this community. A special shout-out to Erica Elliott, Carmen Maendel, Sylvia Becker-Hill, JoAnn Nider, and Amie Rich, who spent a lot of their time sharing their hearts, thoughts, and ideas with me in our group. You all made such an impact on me, completing this book with your encouragement and accountability. I have so much love and appreciation for all of you.

To Katie Shea, you were the spark that got me off the bench with my coaching business journey. The Impact Experience in Chicago was a turning point, where I got out of my own way and began stepping into who I'm meant to be. Your accountability group has been such a significant part of my life, and I am forever grateful to everyone in there. Your beautiful, grounded friendship has been such a blessing. I'm so grateful God crossed our paths.

To Sanjay Raja, and Recipe for Wellness, thank you for believing in me and inviting me to be a part of Season 2 of your incredible show, Recipe for Wellness, on PBS nationwide. Your faith in my message ignited a fire within me to write this book and share it with the world. Because of your support, I wasn't just able to share my story; I was inspired to help create a movement that empowers others to live Unshakable. I'm beyond grateful for your encouragement and belief in what I was called to do.

To my mentors, coaches, and every person who has walked this journey with me: Thank you for your wisdom, your encouragement, and your push to step into my purpose. You have helped me become the woman I am today.

To my family and friends—thank you for seeing me, loving me, and walking beside me on this path. Your encouragement helped me rise again.

To my clients, readers, and every woman and man who has shared their heart with me, you inspire me daily. You remind me why I do this work. Thank you for trusting me with your transformation. It is an honor I do not take lightly.

To my fellow authors, coaches, and collaborators, you've helped me grow, shine, and speak louder. I am grateful to be in your company.

To every woman or man who has ever felt broken, tired, or stuck—I wrote this book for you. I've been where you are. I see you. And I promise you, your story doesn't end here. There is light ahead. And it starts within you.

To the girl I used to be, thank you for not giving up. Thank you for rising when it felt impossible. You were always stronger than you realized. I'm so proud of you.

And finally, to the future version of me who dared to write this book, share her heart, and lead with purpose—thank you for saying yes. You made this real. You made this matter.

This book is not just a project. It's a piece of my soul. Thank you, from the deepest place in my heart, for being part of it. To every reader holding this book: This book exists because of you. You are the reason I wrote these words, the reason I poured my heart onto these pages. Thank you for allowing me to be a part of your journey.

You are not alone.

You are not broken.

You are unshakable.

And now?

It's time to rise.

With all my love,
Sonya McDonald

Table of Contents

Foreword

By Hanna Olivas

There are books that inform.

There are books that inspire.

And then there are books that feel like a lifeline, handwritten by someone who's walked through the fire and lived to build a bridge for the rest of us.

This is one of those books.

I remember the first time I met Sonya. It wasn't just her words that struck me, it was her presence. There was a softness, a sincerity, and an undeniable strength that radiated from her. You could tell instantly, this woman had *lived* through things most people wouldn't survive. But instead of letting those battles define her, she *rose* and then she turned her pain into purpose.

What you're holding in your hands is more than a story. It's a blueprint. It's proof that the human spirit can bend without breaking. It's Sonya's heart on every page, and trust me when I say, these pages will change you.

As the CEO of She Rises Studios and the creator of FENIX TV, I've had the honor of working with thousands of women across the globe who are rebuilding their lives, often from places no one else sees. Chronic illness. Invisible pain. Emotional trauma. Spiritual burnout. Fear. Shame. Silence.

And while every woman's story is unique, there's one thing I know for sure, *We are all one moment away from either breaking... or breaking through.*

That's what Sonya captures so beautifully in this book.

She invites you into her darkest moments, not for pity, not for applause, but so you know *you're not alone.* She brings you into the sterile hospital room, the crushing fatigue, the tears no one else saw, and the prayers whispered in the quiet. And then, brick by brick, she shows you how she built herself back, with purpose, power, and a blueprint that you can follow too.

You don't need to have the same diagnosis to feel seen by this book. You don't need to have a chronic illness to feel the ache in these pages. Because what Sonya's really teaching us isn't just about health, it's about *healing.*

It's about unlearning everything you thought you knew about strength.

It's about redefining what it means to thrive in a world that doesn't always slow down when your body demands it.

It's about choosing to rise, even when rising feels impossible.

And let me tell you, Sonya didn't just write a book. She built a movement.

Her 9-pillar Energy Intelligence Method™ isn't a quick fix. It's not a shiny promise or a social media trend. It's *real,* it's rooted, and it's been lived. She walks her talk. She breathes this message. And she teaches from a place of deep integrity because she's walked this road herself.

There's something sacred about a woman who refuses to let her pain be the final word. Who instead turns around, reaches back, and says to the woman behind her: *"I see you. Let me show you the way forward."*

That's exactly who Sonya is.

And that's exactly what this book will do for you.

So, if you're holding this book right now and wondering if it's really possible to reclaim your health, your joy, your energy, and your power, I want to echo what Sonya will tell you on every page.

Yes. It is.

But it won't come from perfection. It won't come from trying to be everything to everyone while you fall apart inside. It will come from pausing. Listening. Choosing again. And letting healing become your new language.

You're not reading this by accident.

You picked this book up for a reason. Maybe you're tired. Maybe you've been silently suffering. Maybe you've been telling yourself, "I'll start caring for myself when life slows down," or "I'll get better once things settle."

Friend, this book is your moment to stop waiting.

Let Sonya's story remind you that it's never too late to heal. It's never too late to begin again. And you are *never* too far gone to reclaim the light inside you.

Whether this is your rock bottom or your comeback season, welcome to your blueprint.

You are not broken. You are not behind.
You are Unshakable.

Let Sonya guide you home to yourself.
I'll be cheering you on every step of the way.

With so much love and fierce belief in your healing,
Hanna Olivas
CEO of She Rises Studios
Creator of the Sheconomy™
Author | Advocate | Voice for the Unstoppable Woman

Editor's Foreword

As an editor, I've come across many kinds of books. Some are simply there to inform, but others, like Unshakable, stay on your mind long after you've read it.

From the beginning, I could tell this book was more than one about healing and health. It's deeper, a lifeline to those who truly need it. For the overwhelmed, the lost, the weighed-down. It's for those facing a diagnosis that could potentially turn their world on its axis, or for those who carry the heaviness of everyday life on their shoulders.

Unshakable is a book revolving around one woman's healing – healing that feels within reach through a path that feels manageable, even on hard days, offering hope that feels real and grounded.

Sonya McDonald writes with her heart on her sleeve. Her words are filled with quiet strength and tenderness that make the reader feel truly seen. Her story is personal while managing to echo many of our own experiences. Each chapter brings clarity, encouragement, and steps that empower when you're exhausted. The journal prompts included at the end of almost every chapter are another thoughtful touch; real tools for real change.

While editing Unshakable, one thought constantly ran through my mind: this book finds you exactly when you need it. And when you do get your hands on it, and you start embarking on the journey that will transform your life, you'll feel as I felt while reading – like someone is gently reaching out, telling you, "You're not alone in this."

Wherever you are on your life's journey, I hope these pages remind you that healing is possible; it may even be unfolding already.

Sincerely,
Jhan Ellyza Dimatera
SheRisesStudios Publishing Team Editor

Foreword

By Jennifer Jaskal

From the moment I started to read Sonya McDonald's book, "Unshakable: Unlocking Your Blueprint to Living Well Despite Limitations", I was captivated and didn't want to put the book down. Her rawness, authenticity, and vulnerability were refreshing as she wore her heart on her sleeve with every word. Sonya just didn't write about her story; she provides others with tools they are able to implement to turn their life around.

Sonya provides a simple, easy, and effective approach for people to transform their lives. She provides a blueprint for them to take actionable steps; her **R.I.S.E Code™** is easy to remember, and so is her **IGNITE Tool™,** which can help anyone, even children, in 60 seconds to have an energy reset and get back into the moment. These tools are impactful and easy to use on a regular basis.

No matter what you are facing, Sonya helps you to be able to see pieces of yourself in her story through the pain, the fight, the decision to transform her life, and she gives you the ignition for change and to cultivate resilience.

While I was reading, I could see the type of person Sonya is as a loving, caring, and compassionate woman who is here to make a difference in the world. She is not only a magnificent writer; she is a phenomenal woman, speaker, and transformational coach. When you're in her presence, Sonya makes you feel seen and heard, and that's exactly what this book did for me. I was able to see and hear her story, but learn from her that the healing process is a journey and there is no destination. Rather, we can continue on this journey of healing and use these tools to help us become fearless and resilient.

I am so grateful that Sonya was able to share her story and provide others with an opportunity to be the owners of their transformation.

Thank you, Sonya, for all you have done and are doing to help others in their own journeys and in your incredible work.

Sincerely,
Jennifer Jaskal
Leadership Coach | Speaker | Author
CEO & Founder, Jennifer Jaskal, LLC

Foreword

By Erica Elliott

Having had the privilege of reading Sonya McDonald's incredible book, "Unshakable," I can confidently say that it is a captivating read that keeps you on the edge of your seat, making it nearly impossible to put the book down.

Sonya excels at presenting a simple yet profoundly effective approach to transforming your life. She offers a clear blueprint of actionable steps that resonate with anyone seeking change. Her **R.I.S.E. Code™** is a remarkable tool that makes it easy to remember how to rise up with resilience, empowering readers to embrace their strength and overcome challenges.

Throughout the book, Sonya provides a true roadmap to health and well-being, no matter the circumstances one might face. She brings us back to the basics while nurturing a deep love for life, encouraging us to reconnect with what truly matters.

Beyond her writing, Sonya is a phenomenal speaker, seamlessly blending her expertise as a nurse with her knowledge as a transformational coach. Her authentic love for people shines through in her work, and she commands any room she enters with her impactful, glowing presence.

As a counselor, I would highly recommend "Unshakable" to anyone looking to ignite change and cultivate resilience. This book is not just a read; it's a transformative experience that inspires readers to take charge of their lives. Thank you, Sonya, for your incredible work!

Sincerely,

Erica Elliott, MSCP, LPC, CHIMP, CTT, CTFT

Owner of WarriorHeart Healing Hearts, LLC

Foreword

By Kristen Henry

"Unshakable" is a powerful resource for those who often push too hard through the stressors of modern life, ignoring the warning signs that lead to burnout and chronic manifestations.

Sonya shares her deeply personal journey as a busy mom, wife, and nurse, ultimately forced to make a change when her body finally said, 'Enough.' Through her own triumph and clinical background, she shares her blueprint for reflection and recovery, empowering readers with practical tools, promoting true, lasting self-rehabilitation, even when the path feels overwhelming.

Her story is both a wake-up call and a source of hope for anyone seeking holistic healing and balance of the physical, mental, and spiritual being.

The pages in this book remind us that healing is not only possible but essential.

Sincerely,
Kristen Henry, CRDH

Preface

For thirteen years, the relentless grip of Rheumatoid Arthritis and Fibromyalgia dictated my life. The pain was a constant companion, a shadow that never left my side.

Medication became a crutch, offering temporary relief but leaving me with a host of debilitating side effects. Conventional medical approaches felt like a battle I was destined to lose.

I felt the crushing weight of chronic illness, its relentless grip seeping into every corner of my life, threatening to suffocate my spirit. The loneliness was profound, the isolation was crushing.

The pandemic's arrival only intensified my existing struggles; the forced isolation of lockdown became a turning point, a testing ground where I was forced to confront not only my physical limitations but also the deeper emotional wounds that had festered for years.

Yet, within that turning point, a profound transformation began to take shape.

This book isn't just a reflection of my struggles; it's a testament to the power of resilience, the transformative potential of self-discovery, and the unwavering strength of the human spirit.

It's a roadmap to healing, a beacon of hope for others navigating the complex landscape of chronic illness, offering practical strategies and a renewed perspective to help you reclaim your health and well-being.

It's a journey of hope, healing, and rediscovering a life brimming with purpose and joy.

It's a story of hope and transformation, offering inspiration and practical advice to anyone facing health challenges.

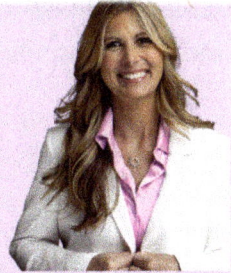

" Your challenges
don't define you.
What you choose
to do with them
does.

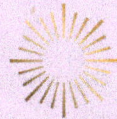

Sonya McDonald
Transformational Life Coach, RN, BSN, BCC

CHAPTER 1

The Moment I Awakened

I could barely breathe. Every inhale felt like dragging air through a straw, my chest tightening as if an invisible force was crushing me from the inside. I was gasping, desperate for oxygen, desperate for relief, but none came.

The car ride to the hospital was a blur. I remember gripping the steering wheel, my knuckles white, my heart pounding harder than my labored breaths. Feverish and drenched in sweat, I stumbled into the hospital, gasping for air that seemed just out of reach.

Nurses rushed to my side, their faces masks of urgent concern, as they wheeled me into the depths of the emergency room. Machines beeped frantically, echoing the chaos in my mind as I realized the gravity of my situation.

In that moment, the harsh reality hit me: I might not make it out of here alive.

Once in the emergency room, the medical staff assessed my condition with swift precision. They placed me in a double isolation room, the result of a new protocol due to the outbreak of a mysterious virus that was spreading globally: COVID-19.

The room was bare and sterile, its walls a blinding white that seemed to absorb all sense of comfort and warmth. The air was thick with the scent of disinfectant, a constant reminder of the invisible threat lurking around every corner. The double isolation measures meant that I was completely cut off from the outside world. No visitors were allowed; not even my closest family members could be by my side.

The door to my room remained closed, a barrier that seemed to solidify my growing sense of isolation. The only human contact I had was with the medical staff, who entered my room in full protective gear, their faces hidden behind masks, shields, and gowns. The anonymity of their appearance made the experience even more surreal and unsettling.

Days stretched into an eternity as I lay in that isolation room, battling the unrelenting fever and struggling to breathe. The ceiling became my canvas, a blank expanse where my mind projected fears and memories. The constant beeping of the heart monitor and the hiss of the breathing treatments were my only companions, their sounds both a comfort and a torment.

Each cough racked my body with pain, my lungs burning with each labored breath. The beeping of monitors, the sterile white walls, the coolness of the IV in my veins, all blurred together into something that felt surreal. But there was nothing surreal about the way my body was betraying me.

This wasn't my Rheumatoid Arthritis. This was something different, something terrifying.

I was locked away in a hospital room, sealed off from the world. No visitors. No family. Just me, the machines, and the gnawing fear that this was it. I had fought so many battles with my body before. But this time, I didn't know if I would win.

The absence of visitors made the experience even more distressing. I longed for the familiar faces of my loved ones, for the comfort of their touch and the sound of their voices. The phone calls and video chats, while a lifeline, could not bridge the gap of physical presence. The isolation weighed heavily on my spirit, amplifying my fears and uncertainties about my outcome.

The nights stretched endlessly. Lying in that bed, I could feel the weight of every moment pressing down on me. The machines beeped rhythmically, an eerie lullaby in the silence. I could hear the nurses whispering outside my door, their hushed voices a reminder that I was being closely watched. Every breath was a fight, and yet, it was in those long, solitary hours that something inside me shifted.

Each passing day felt like a battle fought in solitude, my resilience tested in ways I had never imagined, like a candle's flame enduring the passage of time, its unwavering glow a testament to inner strength.

In the depths of my despair, I turned to prayer. I started praying harder than I ever had before. Not just for healing, but for clarity, for understanding, for strength. I wasn't just asking to be saved, I was asking for a reason to keep fighting. I begged for something to hold onto, something to push me through the fear and exhaustion.

Alone in the sterile isolation room, I prayed to God for strength and guidance. The act of praying provided a sense of peace, a feeling that I was not entirely alone. I poured out my fears, my hopes, and my determination to survive.

In those moments of prayer, I felt a flicker of hope ignite within me, a reminder that there was still something to fight for. Then, a miracle happened.

The hospital made an exception, allowing my daughter to visit me. It was on her Birthday.

She entered the room, gowned and masked, her eyes filled with concern and love. They were pools of compassion reflecting the depths of her love. With each glance, her eyes whispered words of encouragement, painting pictures of healing and strength.

Seeing her was like the sun breaking through the clouds, its rays casting warmth and hope into every corner of my soul. The physical presence of seeing her was an indescribable gift.

Her visit became a turning point in my life. It reignited my will to fight, to get better, to leave that hospital room and return to my life at home with my family, whom I loved and missed so very deeply. This was my awakening moment within. I did not want to just survive this; I wanted to truly live.

The Moment You Realize You Can't Keep Living This Way

Maybe you've never been in a hospital room, hooked up to machines, wondering if you'd make it out alive.

But maybe you have felt trapped in your own body.

Maybe you've had moments where you felt like life was slipping away from you, where fear took over and whispered that you weren't strong enough to fight back. Maybe you've felt like you were just existing, not truly living.

I know what that feels like. I've been there. And if you're reading this, maybe part of you has too.

Here's the truth no one likes to talk about: sometimes, we don't realize how much fear has controlled us until we're staring at the walls of the life it built around us.

I didn't see it clearly until I was lying in that hospital bed. I had spent years living in survival mode. Adapting. Adjusting. Convincing myself that I was fine when, deep down, I was exhausted from the fight.

And maybe that's where you are now. Maybe you've been pushing through, telling yourself you're okay when deep down, you're anything but.

Here's what I need you to understand: you don't have to wait until you're fighting for your life to decide to truly live.

Because that moment will come. Whether it's in a hospital room, in the middle of a breakdown, or staring at yourself in the mirror, wondering where the person you used to be went.

But you don't have to wait until you're at your breaking point. You can decide right now.

The Path to Becoming Unshakable

There comes a moment when you must decide:

Are you going to keep surviving, or are you going to fight for more?

Lying in that hospital bed, I had two choices. I could let fear take over, accept that my body was breaking down, and just exist, trapped in limitations.

Or I could fight.

I could choose to live, not just survive.

Not because it was easy. Not because I suddenly had all the answers. But because I wasn't ready to let my story end there.

And neither are you.

Maybe you've been carrying your own battles, chronic illness, invisible illness, physical or mental trauma, exhaustion, or fear of not being enough. Maybe you've been waiting for something outside of you to change so you can finally start living.

But what if the real change happens inside, you first?

Here's what I want you to know: you are not defined by your diagnosis. You are not defined by your setbacks. You are not defined by your fears.

You are unshakable.

And this book? This journey? It's about unlocking that part of you.

Because if I could come back from that hospital room, weak, exhausted, and afraid, and build a life of purpose and strength, then so can you.

Journal Prompt: Unlocking Your Own Awakening

Take a deep breath. Now, grab a journal and answer this:

1. Where in my life have I been "just surviving" instead of truly living?
2. What fears have been holding me back from stepping fully into my power?
3. What is one small action I can take today to start living differently?

_____

_____

_____

_____

_____

_____

_____

_____

_____

_____

_____

_____

_____

_____

Final Words

This was my awakening. The moment I chose to fight back instead of letting my fears, my illness, and my circumstances dictate my life.

In Chapter 2, we're going back, back to where it all started. To the moment I was diagnosed with Rheumatoid Arthritis, to the fear that started creeping in long before that hospital room.

Are you ready? Let's go.

The Moment Everything Changed

I still remember the moment my world shifted. I want you to imagine being 36 years old, standing in the Florida sun at SeaWorld, and there is not a cloud in the sky. You hear the sound of roller coasters rushing past, the scent of popcorn, cinnamon rolls, French fries, and sunscreen in the air. Laughter echoes from families all around you.

You're pushing a stroller, your little one nestled inside, while your other daughter is skipping ahead with her dad and grandparents, giggling, carefree. It's supposed to be a perfect day. A day of creating beautiful memories. Then, in a split second, everything changes.

You look down at your hands. They have doubled in size, and you can't make a fist. You lose your grasp of the stroller. Your fingers are tingling, and it feels as if bees are stinging you all over. You lose your grip on the stroller, and you can't make a fist.

You try to tighten your hold, but your hands won't listen.

Your knees lock up. Your ankles weld together. Each step feels like you're walking through wet cement. Your body is shutting down, and you don't know why.

Panic sets in.

What's happening to me?

Your children are still laughing, still running ahead, but you? You're frozen.

A wave of terror crashes over you.

No warning. No time to prepare.

Your life, everything you've ever known, just changed in an instant.

That was my reality.

But what about you?

Have you ever had a moment where everything shifted?

Where one piece of news, one bad day, one diagnosis, one failure, one unexpected twist—changed everything?

Have you ever felt like life just pulled the rug out from under you and left you standing there, wondering what now?

For me, I had always been the woman who kept going, pushing through no matter what. I ignored the signs, telling myself just one more thing, I'll rest later. But my body kept the score. It had its own warning system, and when I ignored it for too long, it hit the red light, and it shut down completely.

Have you ever ignored the warning signs? Do you push through exhaustion? You tell yourself to rest later. You think you can handle it all until suddenly your body, your mind, or your life throws up a red light you just can't ignore.

> *"We don't lose ourselves all at once;*
> *we lose ourselves one small sacrifice at a time."*

The Diagnosis That Changed Everything

Not long after, I sat in a doctor's office, waiting for answers.

And then came the words that changed everything:

"Sonya, you have Rheumatoid Arthritis and Fibromyalgia."

And before I could even process those words, the doctor continued:

"You'll be in a wheelchair within six months if you don't start the medications immediately."

"You won't be able to have any more children."

"You need to start medication immediately, and that means no more breastfeeding. Stop today."

That was it.

No discussion. No choice.

I sat there, holding my baby, feeling like my body had just betrayed me. Those words the doctor said hung in the air, heavy and suffocating, like a physical weight pressing down on my chest.

One moment, I was a whirlwind of activity, a Registered nurse, a devoted wife, a mom juggling career, family, and the joys of everyday life. I was the woman who could do it all.

Now? I was the patient. Now, the future stretched before me, an uncertain and terrifying landscape of pain, limitations, and uncertainty. The diagnosis wasn't just a medical label; it was a death sentence to the life I knew.

The strong, unstoppable woman I once knew was gone.

And fear took over like nothing I have ever felt before.

Have you ever felt like your whole identity was ripped away in an instant?

Like everything you worked for, built, dreamed of, was suddenly no longer possible?

Maybe for you, it wasn't a diagnosis.

Maybe it was a job loss. Maybe it was a divorce. Maybe it was the loss of someone you love. Maybe it was standing in front of a mirror, realizing you didn't even recognize yourself anymore.

Have you ever felt like life just handed you a script you never asked for, and now you don't even know what role you're playing anymore?

"Fear doesn't protect you; it paralyzes you."

Living in Fear – Surviving, Not Living

For the next 13 years, I didn't live; I survived.

I was trapped.

Trapped in fear of germs, sickness, and setbacks.

Trapped in fear of what my body could no longer do.

Trapped in the belief that my life was over before it had even really begun.

I had to cut back on my work as a nurse because exhaustion made it impossible for me to stand through shifts.

Isolation became a constant companion, deepening as the relentless fatigue made it difficult to maintain my social connections.

Friends and acquaintances drifted away, their lives continuing while mine seemed to be permanently stalled. The social activities that once brought joy and fulfillment were no longer accessible, leaving me feeling increasingly disconnected and alone. Even maintaining basic relationships became an insurmountable struggle as my ability to participate was limited by the pain and fatigue. The joy I found in helping others, a keystone in my life as a registered nurse, was forever lost under the heavy weight of my health struggles.

The emotional toll on my family was immeasurable. They watched helplessly as I battled my illness, their lives indirectly impacted by the daily struggles I faced. Their support was unwavering, but the constant strain of my condition weighed heavily on all of us. The unspoken anxieties and shared worries cast a long shadow over our once vibrant family life. I felt guilty for the burden I placed on my loved ones, for the ways my illness affected their daily routines and peace of mind. The silent struggles we all endured were a testament to the profound and far-reaching effects of chronic illness.

I felt like a broken record, repeating my story of pain and limitation to doctors, friends, and family alike. Their sympathy, while well-intentioned, didn't alleviate the pain that consumed my every waking moment. The feeling of being misunderstood, of being invisible behind the mask of my chronic illness, intensified my isolation.

The pain and fatigue made social interactions difficult, forcing me to withdraw from friends and activities I once cherished.

The vibrant life I once knew faded into a muted existence, confined to the four walls of my home. The joy I once found in my work as a nurse and the satisfaction of caring for others were replaced by a crushing self-consciousness and physical limitations. My inability to perform even the simplest tasks, like opening a jar or brushing my hair, fueled a deep sense of inadequacy and self-doubt.

The seemingly effortless lives of others became a constant source of frustration, a brutal contrast to my own limited existence. I longed for the days when I could easily walk my dog, visit friends, or engage in the activities that once filled my days with joy. Instead, I was trapped in a world of pain, unable to participate in the activities that gave my life meaning and purpose.

This feeling of being trapped in a body that was no longer my own, coupled with the constant pain and debilitating fatigue, led to a deep sense of hopelessness.

I questioned the meaning of my existence, wondering if this was all there was, a life defined by pain and limitation. The future seemed bleak, an endless expanse of suffering with no escape in sight. Even the smallest tasks seemed monumental, my spirit worn down by the relentless battle against my own body.

It was during this period, in the quiet despair of my own home, that I began to question everything, my purpose, my identity, and my future. The crushing weight of my diagnosis threatened to extinguish the very spark of life within me.

The emotional toll was as devastating as the physical pain. Depression crept in, wrapping around my heart, suffocating my hopes and dreams. The darkness was absolute. It wasn't the darkness of a moonless night, but a darkness that resided within, a suffocating blanket woven from pain, fatigue, and despair.

For thirteen years, I had navigated the treacherous terrain of Rheumatoid Arthritis and Fibromyalgia, clinging to the hope that a cure, a miracle, would emerge from the fog of treatments and medications. But the hope, once a beacon, had dwindled to a flickering candle flame, threatened constantly by the winds of disappointment.

Anxiety became a constant companion, its icy grip tightening its hold whenever I tried to push myself beyond my physical limits. The relentless cycle of pain, medication, and exhaustion eroded my sense of self-worth, leaving me feeling helpless and utterly alone. I was desperately seeking a way out of the darkness, a beacon of hope in the seemingly endless tunnel of suffering.

It was a dark and desperate time, but unbeknownst to me, it was also the darkest hour before dawn. The seeds of transformation were quietly being sown, even in the depths of my despair.

The initial wave of medications prescribed felt like a lifeline, a desperate grab for normalcy in a sea of pain. Methotrexate, prednisone, and steroid injections and a cocktail of NSAIDs became my daily companions, their promises of relief often overshadowed by their harsh realities. The nausea was relentless, a constant churning in my stomach that left me weak and depleted. The dizziness made even the simplest tasks feel like navigating a tilting ship, a constant threat of imbalance and falls. And the fatigue...oh, the fatigue. It was an oppressive weight, a heavy blanket smothering my energy, leaving me drained and listless. I spent many days simply existing, a shadow of my former self, struggling to perform even basic self-care.

The physical therapy sessions were equally challenging. The exercises, designed to improve my range of motion and strengthen my weakened muscles, often left me in excruciating pain. Each session was a grueling battle against my own body, a testament to the limitations my illness imposed. The therapists, kind and compassionate though they were, couldn't erase the deep-seated pain that pulsed through my joints and muscles. Their encouragement felt hollow, a fragile counterpoint to the overwhelming despair that often consumed me.

My days were a monotonous cycle of medication, therapy, and rest, punctuated by frequent trips to various specialists. Rheumatologists, gastroenterologists, neurologists – each appointment offered a fleeting glimmer of hope, a new diagnosis, a new medication, a new treatment plan. But each new hope soon faded into disillusionment as the pain remained stubbornly resistant to every intervention. Each consultation felt like a gamble, a desperate roll of the dice in a game I felt destined to lose.

The emotional toll was just as profound. The lack of progress fueled a deep sense of hopelessness. My self-esteem plummeted, replaced by a gnawing sense of inadequacy and self-doubt. I felt like a broken machine, beyond repair, destined for a life of pain and limitation. The vibrant, energetic woman I once was seemed like a distant memory, a ghost of my past self.

I truly was not living as my old unstoppable self. I was living in such a great amount of fear.

I spent my life avoiding, shrinking, and fearing the next flare-up.

I told myself:

"If I can just make it through today..."

"If I can just get by..."

But tell me—how many of you have said those exact words to yourself?

"If I can just make it to the weekend."

"If I can just hold it together a little longer."

"If I can just survive this season of life."

But here's the truth.

You weren't made to just survive, you were made to THRIVE.

That pain was the beginning of everything.

And I had no idea that day at SeaWorld would mark the moment my life would never be the same again.

What Fear Is Controlling Your Life?

I wonder, what are you afraid of? Because fear doesn't just show up in the obvious ways. It disguises itself as logic. As a responsibility. As self-protection.

But in reality?

Fear is a cage.

And if you're not careful, it will shrink your world down to nothing.

For 13 years, I let fear dictate my choices:

- I stopped traveling because I was afraid I wouldn't be able to handle the exhaustion.
- I stopped going on hikes or long walks because I was afraid my joints would flare up.
- I stopped saying yes to things that brought me joy, because I was too scared of what might happen if I did.

What about you? Where has fear been making your decisions for you?

Because here's the truth: if you don't face it, fear will keep you stuck. It will convince you that playing small is the safest option.

But it's not. It's just a slow form of disappearing.

The Truth That Set Me Free

I wish I could tell you I realized this sooner.

But the truth is that it took 13 years before I finally saw what fear had done to me.

I had lived in survival mode for so long that I had forgotten what it felt like to truly live.

And it all came crashing down in March of 2020, when I ended up in the hospital, gasping for breath.

That was my breaking point.

That was when I knew I couldn't keep living like this. Something had to change.

And that's when I started building the blueprint that changed my life.

The Decision That Changed Everything

The moment I left the hospital, I made a choice.

I was done being afraid.

I was done waiting for my body to fail me.

I was done letting fear control me.

I didn't want to just survive. I wanted to live.

And that meant I had to do something I had never done before: I had to take control of my own health.

Not just my physical health, but my mental, emotional, and spiritual health, too.

For the first time in 13 years, I asked myself: "What if I stopped making decisions based on fear? What if I built a life that actually helped me thrive, despite my diagnosis?"

And that's exactly what I did.

Deciding to stop living in fear was the first step.

But the next step?

I needed a plan.

A system.

A way to actually live well despite my diagnosis.

And that's where the blueprint comes in.

Because Here's What I Know

Fear will keep you stuck for as long as you let it.

But the moment you decide to break free?

Everything changes.

In Chapter 3, I'll show you exactly how I did it. Because you don't just break free from fear, you build a life beyond it.

And that's where we're going next.

Journal Prompt: Facing Your Fear

Take a moment to reflect. Grab a journal and answer these questions honestly:

1. What is one thing fear has been keeping you from?
2. What would your life look like if you weren't afraid?
3. What is one small step you can take today to start reclaiming your power?
4. If you stopped living in survival mode, what would you do differently?

_____

_____

_____

_____

_____

_____

_____

_____

_____

_____

_____

_____

CHAPTER 3

The Unshakable Blueprint – The 9 Pillars of The Energy Intelligence Method™

When everything in my life came crashing down, my health, my energy, my sense of self, I had no idea how I'd rebuild. I just knew I couldn't go back to the way things were. The hospital bed I found myself in 2020 wasn't just a medical crisis; it was an awakening. I had been given a second chance, and I was not going to waste it. I couldn't outrun my pain anymore. I had to face it, feel it, and find a new way to live.

The initial days were consumed by fear and anxiety, but gradually, a different kind of energy began to emerge. It was a quieter, more inward-focused energy – a space for self-reflection that had been previously unavailable. Confined to my home, I had time to observe my body, listen to its subtle cues, and pay attention to the ways in which my lifestyle choices were either contributing to or exacerbating my pain and fatigue.

The journey from the darkest hour to the dawn of recovery was not easy, but it was a journey worth taking. It was a journey of self-discovery, of resilience, of transformation. And it is a journey that I am eager to share with you who are struggling with invisible chronic illnesses and other challenges and limitations.

For those who feel the weight of their condition is an insurmountable burden, I offer hope. It's possible to move from a place of despair to one of discovery; it's possible to reclaim your life and find a way to thrive, even amidst pain and suffering.

My path may not be yours, but the lessons learned resonate universally: hope can be found in the darkest hours, resilience is possible even when facing the most challenging circumstances, and the power to shape your own life remains even when health limitations are present. The key is to recognize your own strength and to embark on that journey, one step at a time, one breath at a time.

Being in the hospital in 2020, when the world as we knew it had shut down for quite some time, there was so much fear along with the uncertainty of the pandemic all around. I knew the feeling all too well, living in fear for the past 13 years. There were a lot of adaptations after I went home from the hospital and I had to start slow in my recovery.

The pandemic, a period initially characterized by fear and uncertainty, ultimately became a catalyst for profound personal growth and transformation. It forced me to confront the realities of my chronic illnesses in a way that I had never done before, to re-evaluate my priorities, and to commit to a path of wellness that was both holistic and sustainable.

The pandemic forced a radical shift in my perspective. The world, once perceived as a relentless, demanding force outside my control, became a space of opportunity, of introspection, of self-discovery. The threat of the virus, though terrifying, ignited a fire within me – a renewed commitment to my health, my well-being, and my own resilience.

The forced slowdown was a period of intense self-examination that led to a profound transformation in my understanding of myself and my illness. It was a time of deep introspection, a period of peeling back layers of denial and self-neglect, and of embracing a journey of self-discovery that ultimately sparked lasting change in every corner of my life.

The isolation initially felt stifling, a prison of my own making. But over time, this isolation became a sanctuary, a place of refuge where I could focus on my internal world, unburdened by the external demands that had once defined my existence. The solitude allowed me to connect with myself on a deeper level than ever before. I began to understand the subtle nuances of my body's responses to stress, to pain, and to the various treatments I had undergone over the years.

I discovered the importance of self-compassion, a quality I had previously lacked. The pandemic, in its cruel irony, provided a context in which self-criticism felt almost unbearable. The constant threat of illness and death forced me to recognize my own fragility, to acknowledge my vulnerabilities without judgment. This, in turn, allowed me to cultivate a more nurturing and understanding relationship with myself – a shift in perspective that proved crucial in my journey towards healing.

It was in those moments of quiet reflection, amidst the fear and uncertainty, that I began to truly understand the power of self-love, self-acceptance, and self-compassion.

The journey was far from easy, but the lessons learned were invaluable. It was a journey that taught me the importance of self-care, self-compassion, and the power of resilience in the face of adversity. It was a journey that ultimately led me to a deeper understanding of myself and my capacity for healing, both physically and emotionally.

Within the four walls of my home, I began to feel a power shift. It wasn't a dramatic moment of empowerment, but rather a quiet, internal revolution. The realization that I held the power to shape my life and control my response to my circumstances began to take root. The external chaos, the constant threat of infection and mortality, forced me to confront the ultimate reality: my life was precious, and it was my responsibility to honor and protect it.

This wasn't about denying the reality of my illnesses. It wasn't about pretending that the pain and fatigue disappeared overnight. It was about acknowledging those realities and actively choosing to respond to them in a way that empowered me, rather than allowing them to diminish me. It was about seizing control of my narrative and writing a new chapter in the story of my life.

The simple act of conscious breathing created a space between the pain and my reaction to it. It gave me a moment of peace, a brief pause from the overwhelming sense of helplessness. And in that moment, I recognized a profound truth: even in the midst of intense physical suffering, I had the power to choose my response. I could choose to give in to despair, or I could choose to find strength, resilience, and hope.

This realization was transformative. It shifted the balance of power from my illnesses to me. It didn't erase the pain, but it diminished its power over my spirit. It empowered me to take active steps to manage my symptoms, to advocate for my needs, and to create a life that was fulfilling despite the limitations imposed by my chronic conditions.

This journey of empowerment wasn't linear. There were setbacks, moments of doubt, and times when the old patterns of passivity threatened to reassert themselves. But with each setback, I learned to recognize the power of choice, to consciously select a response that aligned with my values, my goals, and my desire for a life of meaning and purpose. I learned to celebrate small victories, to acknowledge the progress made, even amidst the challenges.

My home, once a sanctuary from the demands of the outside world, had now become a laboratory for self-discovery. It was within those walls that I began to meticulously track my symptoms, to identify triggers, and to experiment with different strategies for managing my health. I became my own researcher, my own advocate, my own healer.

I revisited the holistic approaches I had dabbled in before—mindfulness, meditation, nutritional changes, and gentle movement—with renewed focus.

For 13 years, I had lived in fear of my body, of pain, of getting worse. I had let my illness control me, making decisions based on what I was afraid might happen instead of what I actually wanted.

But that hospital stay was my wake-up call.

I had been given a second chance, and I wasn't going to waste it.

I had spent my career as a nurse, helping others take care of their bodies. Now, I had to turn that knowledge inward.

I had to build a blueprint, a system, a structure, a way to actually live well despite my diagnosis and any limitations I may face.

No more waiting.

No more playing small.

No more fear.

It was time to take control of my life.

And that's exactly what I did.

The First Step: Redefining Health

Before I could make any real changes, I had to unlearn everything I thought I knew about health.

For years, I had believed that health was just about fixing symptoms.

If I was in pain? Take medication.

If I was exhausted? Drink more coffee.

If I was overwhelmed? Push through.

But none of that was actually healing me.

True health wasn't just about treating the body.

It was about aligning the mind, body, and spirit.

For the first time in my life, I stopped asking, How do I make this pain go away?

And I started asking, How do I create a life that supports my healing?

What's Your Definition of Health?

I want you to take a moment and ask yourself:

What does "being healthy" actually mean to you?

Not what society says.

Not what your doctors have told you.

Not what you used to believe.

But you.

Because here's the truth,

Most of us have been taught a very narrow version of health.

We think it means:

- Losing weight
- Taking medication
- Exercising until we're exhausted
- Eating salads and drinking water

But real health?

It's so much bigger than that.

Health is about energy.

Health is about clarity.

Health is about peace.

And until you define what health actually means to you, you'll never fully claim it.

So, what does it look like for you?

That was the moment I began asking new questions:

"What if healing wasn't just about getting rid of symptoms?"

"What if I could live well even while still managing illness?"

"What if I was never meant to go back to who I was... but forward into who I was becoming?"

And most of all...

"What if I could become unshakable, not because I was never shaken, but because I learned how to rise, again and again?"

That question changed everything. This is when I began to build my blueprint for living well despite any limitations.

And from that moment forward, I started building a new foundation, not just for healing, but for thriving. Through every breakdown, every setback, every breakthrough, I discovered nine essential pillars that became the core of my transformation. These were not trends, quick fixes, or magic answers. They were grounded, intentional, and deeply personal.

This is the blueprint that helped me get my life back.

And it's the same framework I now teach to women around the world who are ready to reclaim theirs.

The Unshakable Blueprint – The 9 Pillars of the Energy Intelligence Method™

This is the structure I return to again and again. These nine pillars helped me rise from my lowest point and are the very heartbeat of how I live today:

1. Fuel Your Body for Healing - Food is Medicine
2. Master Your Mindset
3. Move Your Body with Love
4. Connect to Faith and Purpose
5. Protect Your Energy and Set Empowered Boundaries (**The IGNITE Tool™**)
6. Rise with Resilience (**The R.I.S.E. Code™**)

7. Heal Through Love, Forgiveness, and Emotional Freedom
8. Leading with Purpose (Share your light and serve from the Heart)
9. Tiny Habits Lead to Big Change

Each pillar plays a crucial role in your healing and your transformation.

In the following chapters, I will go deeper into all nine pillars of my blueprint journey and transformation. For now, let me walk you through what each one means.

Pillar 1: Fuel Your Body for Healing – Food is Medicine

When I was first diagnosed with Rheumatoid Arthritis and Fibromyalgia, I tried everything the medical system offered—medications, treatments, and symptom management. But deep down, I knew healing had to start from the inside.

I had to change the way I was fueling my body.

And no, I don't just mean food. Yes, anti-inflammatory nutrition played a huge role. I started drinking celery juice daily, reducing processed foods, and learning what made my body feel good rather than inflamed.

But fuel also meant hydration, supplements, rest, breath, joy, laughter, and emotional nourishment.

It meant asking: "What am I feeding myself in every area of my life?"

Fueling my body became a form of love. I wasn't punishing it anymore. I was honoring it.

This pillar is about treating your body as the sacred vessel it is, not waiting until it breaks down, but learning how to pour into it daily.

Pillar 2: Master Your Mindset

You can't heal a body you hate. And you can't change your life while thinking the same thoughts that got you stuck in the first place.

Mindset is everything.

I spent years stuck in fear. Fear of pain. Fear of losing control. Fear of being a burden. Fear of not being enough.

But I didn't realize that my thoughts were shaping my reality. They were influencing my decisions, my mood, my energy, and even my pain.

I had to learn how to rewrite the stories in my head—how to challenge the inner critic, speak truth over my life, and choose hope over despair.

This is where journaling became my lifeline.

Gratitude journaling. Rewriting my beliefs. Visualizing healing. Speaking affirmations out loud.

I stopped saying things like "I'm broken" and started declaring, "I'm healing."

I stopped asking "Why me?" and started asking, "What now?"

This pillar helped me rebuild my identity from the inside out. And when you master your mindset, nothing can steal your peace.

Pillar 3: Move Your Body with Love

For years, I equated movement with punishment. I believed if I wasn't working out hard, I wasn't doing enough. But with chronic illness, that mindset only led to more pain, more guilt, more shame.

I had to redefine movement.

Not as something I "had" to do, but something I got to do.

Some days looked like a walk in nature. Other days, it meant gentle stretching or dancing in the kitchen. The key was learning to listen to my body, not override it.

I started asking myself: "What movement would feel like love today?"

Movement became less about fitness and more about freedom. It helped me reconnect with my body in a way that was kind, joyful, and safe. I didn't need to push—I just needed to be present.

This pillar is not about intensity. It's about intention. It's about celebrating what your body can do, not punishing it for what it can't.

Pillar 4: Connect to Faith and Purpose

There were moments on this journey when nothing made sense. The pain. The loss. The fear. And in those moments, the only thing I had left to hold onto was my faith.

When the world goes quiet, and you're left in the stillness of your struggle, faith becomes your anchor.

But it wasn't just about faith—it was about reconnecting with my purpose.

I believe each of us was created with something inside that the world needs. When we align with our purpose, even the pain starts to make sense. My struggles became my calling. My healing became my mission.

This pillar reminds you that you're not here by accident. You're not broken. You're being shaped for impact, for transformation, for something greater than yourself.

Faith and purpose breathe life back into you when you feel lost. They lift your eyes off your circumstances and remind you who you are and whose you are.

Pillar 5: Protect Your Energy and Set Empowered Boundaries (The IGNITE Tool™)

I created **THE IGNITE Tool™: Your 60-Second Energy Reset** for those who need to reset and shift their energy in 60 seconds. It's a tool to help you go from being overwhelmed or emotionally dysregulated to calm and focused.

This one changed everything.

Because no matter how much healing work I did, if I was still overextending, people-pleasing, and tolerating what drained me, I would end up back in burnout.

Your energy is sacred. Boundaries protect it.

I had to learn to say no. To cancel plans. To listen when my body said "not today." I had to walk away from toxic dynamics and unlearn the belief that my worth came from being everything to everyone.

Protecting my peace became a daily practice.

And it made every other pillar sustainable.

Boundaries are not about pushing people away; they're about keeping your healing safe.

This pillar will teach you how to stop leaking energy and start living aligned.

Pillar 6: Rise with Resilience – (The R.I.S.E. Code™)

This pillar is about transforming your setbacks into comebacks.

This blueprint teaches you how to rebuild your strength from within, rise above fear, and stand tall in the face of adversity by following the **R.I.S.E. Code™**—a proven mindset framework rooted in resilience, identity, self-worth, and empowered action.

Pillar 7: Heal Through Love – Forgiveness and Emotional Freedom

This pillar is about unlocking deep healing by choosing love over bitterness and grace over guilt.

This blueprint guides you in forgiving yourself and others, releasing emotional burdens, and stepping into true freedom, where peace, self-compassion, and wholeness begin.

Pillar 8: Lead with Purpose – Share Your Light and Serve from the Heart

This pillar is about turning your healing into purpose.

This blueprint empowers you to rise from what you've overcome, share your story, and make a difference by serving others with authenticity, love, and impact. It's where your transformation becomes someone else's inspiration.

Pillar 9: Tiny Habits Lead to Big Change

Tiny consistent habits over time may seem small, but when repeated daily, they create powerful momentum. One small shift at a time is how big, lasting transformation begins.

The Blueprint That Transforms

Each of these pillars work together like gears in a machine. When one turns, the others start to move. When you fuel your body, your energy improves. When your energy improves, your mindset shifts. When your mindset shifts, you find the strength to rise. When you move with love, you reconnect with faith. When you connect with faith, you find purpose.

When you protect your energy and set empowered boundaries, you create the space to stay aligned with that purpose without burning out.

From that place of grounded strength, you rise with resilience, learning to stand tall through adversity and bounce back stronger every time life tries to knock you down. And as you rise, you're called to let go of what no longer serves you.

Forgiveness and love become the healing balm, setting you free emotionally and spiritually. Once you've healed through love, you're ready for the final gear to turn, stepping fully into your calling. When you lead with purpose and serve from the heart, you become a light for others, showing them what's possible when you choose healing, wholeness, and truth.

But none of that will last unless you protect your energy and hold your boundaries like your peace depends on it.

Because it does.

My Promise to You

You don't need to master all nine pillars overnight.

You just need to begin.

This book will walk you through each one—step by step, with love, grace, and truth. I'll share the blueprint that helped me rise from rock bottom and rebuild a life I love. And I'll give you the tools to do the same.

You may have limitations, but you are not limited.

You may have been shaken, but you are still standing.

And from here on out, you don't just survive.

You become Unshakable.

CHAPTER 4

Pillar 1 – Fuel Your Body for Healing – Food is Medicine

I used to think of food as an afterthought. Something to get through the day, to fix a craving, or to numb the stress I didn't want to feel. I was busy, overwhelmed, exhausted—and like so many women, I put myself last. I grabbed what was convenient, skipped meals, or filled my body with things I thought were "normal," even though they were hurting me.

But my body had been whispering for years. And when I didn't listen, it started screaming.

The pain became impossible to ignore. My joints throbbed. I had brain fog so intense I couldn't form sentences. I was exhausted by noon. I'd cry in the car from pain and frustration, pretending I was okay when I wasn't. Eventually, my body forced me to stop. It forced me to pay attention.

That's when I began to understand something so many of us miss: **Healing begins with how you fuel your body.**

My kitchen, once a battlefield of convenience and quick fixes, was now undergoing a complete transformation. The shelves, once stocked with brightly colored boxes and bags promising instant gratification, were slowly but surely being emptied, replaced with fresh produce, whole grains, and unprocessed ingredients. This wasn't merely a dietary change; it was a complete overhaul of my relationship with food. It was a journey that demanded patience, perseverance, and a willingness to confront deeply ingrained habits.

The initial days were challenging. The cravings hit hard – the salty crunch of potato chips, the sugary sweetness of processed snacks, the comforting familiarity of fast food. My body, accustomed to the processed sugar and refined carbohydrates, rebelled. Headaches, fatigue, and irritability were common companions. I found myself battling intense waves of desire, a physical manifestation of my body's dependence on the very foods I was trying to eliminate.

My initial grocery shopping trips were exercises in self-control. I would meticulously read labels, scrutinizing ingredient lists for hidden sugars, unhealthy fats, and artificial additives. I learned to decipher the nutritional information, understanding serving sizes and caloric values. The experience was often frustrating and time-consuming, but it was also incredibly educational.

The transition from processed foods to whole foods wasn't about deprivation; it was about mindful substitution. Instead of reaching for a bag of chips, I began experimenting with roasted chickpeas, seasoned with herbs and spices. The satisfying crunch satisfied the craving while providing a healthier, nutrient-rich alternative. My sweet cravings were appeased with fresh fruit or a small amount of dark chocolate. The instant gratification of processed snacks was replaced by the slower, more mindful pleasure of preparing and savoring whole foods.

Cooking became a form of self-care. I started experimenting with new recipes, discovering the simple joy of preparing meals from scratch. I found myself drawn to cuisines rich in fresh vegetables, lean proteins, and whole grains. I discovered the subtle flavors of different herbs and spices, as well as the delightful textures of various fruits and vegetables. The act of cooking became a meditative practice, a way to connect with my body and nourish it with wholesome, nourishing foods.

There were setbacks, of course. There were days when I caved in to the temptation of processed foods, moments of weakness where old habits reasserted themselves. But with each setback, I learned to practice self-compassion, acknowledging my imperfections without judgment. I reframed these slips as opportunities for learning, moments to examine my triggers and develop strategies to cope with cravings. I didn't beat myself up; I simply adjusted my approach and continued on my journey.

One of the biggest challenges was managing my cravings for sugar. Processed foods are often loaded with refined sugar, which triggers a cascade of addictive responses in the brain. Eliminating these foods meant confronting my body's dependence on sugar. I experimented with different strategies to manage my cravings, including reducing my overall sugar intake gradually, finding healthy substitutes like fruit or stevia, and staying hydrated. I also discovered the importance of sleep and stress management in curbing sugar cravings.

My kitchen transformed from being a symbol of convenience and instant gratification to a sanctuary of health and well-being. Gone were the processed foods that once lined the shelves; they were now stocked with fresh, vibrant ingredients, reflecting a transformed relationship with food, built on respect, intention, and mindful nourishment. It was a testament to the power of conscious choice, the transformative potential of food, and the unwavering resilience of the human spirit.

Over time, I found ways to enjoy social occasions without compromising my commitment to whole foods. I learned to embrace the challenge of adapting my dietary needs to various social situations, demonstrating a strength of character and resilience that extended far beyond the kitchen. It became a testament to my dedication to my overall well-being, not as a restrictive diet but as a conscious lifestyle choice.

The journey wasn't always smooth sailing. There were moments of doubt, times when I questioned my ability to maintain this new lifestyle. But with each challenge, I developed new strategies and coping mechanisms. I learned to listen to my body's cues, becoming more attuned to its signals of hunger, satiety, and cravings.

The shift in my food choices had a profound impact on my overall health. Not only did my physical symptoms improve, but my mental clarity and emotional stability also benefited greatly. I found myself less susceptible to mood swings and more resilient in the face of stress. The connection between my food choices and my overall well-being became undeniably clear.

The transformation was not merely about eliminating processed foods, but about a fundamental shift in perspective. It was about acknowledging my power to influence my own health and well-being through mindful choices. It was a journey of self-discovery, a testament to the remarkable ability of the human body to heal and thrive when provided with the right nourishment. The kitchen, once a site of struggle, became a laboratory for self-healing and a testament to the powerful connection between food, body, and mind. My relationship with food had changed completely, transforming from a source of fleeting satisfaction to one of sustainable well-being.

My transformation extended beyond simply eliminating processed foods; it delved into the realm of proactive nourishment. I discovered the power of juicing, a daily ritual that became an integral part of my healing journey. The journey of incorporating juicing into my daily routine became a huge part of my overall approach to healing. It was a testament to my resilience, adaptability, and unwavering commitment to nurturing my body and mind. It became an emblem of self-love and acceptance, a daily reminder of the powerful connection between food, health, and overall well-being. The humble act of juicing transformed into a potent symbol of self-empowerment, a daily affirmation of my capacity for self-healing, and a profound act of self-care. This simple ritual resonated far beyond the confines of my kitchen, extending its healing power to every aspect of my life.

My journey toward whole foods wasn't a sudden, dramatic shift but a gradual evolution and a mindful exploration of what truly nourished my body. It began with small changes, subtle substitutions that slowly but surely transformed my dietary landscape.

The transformation started with the fruits and vegetables.

My meals evolved to reflect this new focus on whole foods.

Breakfast, once a rushed affair of sugary cereals or pastries, transformed into a nourishing ritual. A bowl of oatmeal topped with fresh berries and a sprinkle of nuts became my staple, providing sustained energy and a symphony of flavors.

Lunch often consisted of large salads brimming with fresh greens, colorful vegetables, and lean protein sources, like grilled chicken or fish. I discovered the versatility of quinoa, incorporating it into bowls with roasted vegetables, chickpeas, and a light lemon vinaigrette. These meals weren't just fuel; they were a celebration of flavor, color, and nourishment.

Dinner became a culinary adventure, a chance to experiment with new recipes and explore different flavor combinations. I embraced the simplicity of roasted vegetables, experimenting with various herbs and spices to create unique and delicious dishes. Root vegetables, like sweet potatoes and carrots, became my culinary companions, offering a sweetness that satisfied my cravings for sugary treats without the detrimental effects. I learned to appreciate the earthy flavors of mushrooms and the subtle bitterness of broccoli, discovering a palate for tastes I had previously overlooked. Lean protein sources, such as salmon, chicken breast, and lentils, provided the building blocks for muscle repair and overall health.

My exploration extended to the realm of healthy fats, crucial for hormonal balance and cellular function. Avocado became a culinary staple, its creamy texture and rich flavor adding a luxurious touch to salads, sandwiches, and even smoothies. Nuts and seeds, such as almonds, walnuts, chia seeds, and flaxseeds, became regular additions to my meals, providing essential fatty acids and a satisfying crunch. Olive oil replaced less healthy cooking oils, adding a distinctive Mediterranean flair to my culinary creations. I discovered the health benefits of coconut oil and incorporated it into my cooking and skincare routines.

It wasn't just about consuming fruits and vegetables; it was about absorbing their potent life force, a concentrated burst of vitamins, minerals, and enzymes that fueled my body's natural healing capabilities.

The effects were noticeable almost immediately. Celery juicing was the key to reducing my inflammation and helping me heal so much from the inside out. I had no idea how powerful a single vegetable could be—until I discovered celery. It became a daily ritual in my fight against inflammation. I did this with two stalks of celery on an empty stomach every morning upon awakening. Nothing else. I waited 30 minutes before consuming anything else. That simple habit became a game-changer in my Rheumatoid Arthritis and Fibromyalgia journey. I first learned about it from Anthony William's Celery Juice book, which I discovered while attending Tony Robbins' Unleash the Power Within conference. What seemed ordinary turned out to be extraordinary healing from the inside out.

My energy levels surged, a stark contrast to the chronic fatigue I had experienced for so long. My digestion, which had been a source of constant discomfort, improved dramatically. The inflammation that had plagued my body for years began to subside. I felt lighter, more vibrant, and more alive.

I started keeping a detailed journal, documenting my juicing experiments, the ingredient combinations, and their effects on my body. I always stick to my routine, which includes 16 ounces of plain celery juice every morning on an empty stomach, with no additives, followed by at least 30 minutes before introducing any food for the day. After that part of my daily routine, I would enjoy experimenting with juicing other fruits and vegetables. This became a valuable tool, enabling me to track my progress and refine my recipes over time. It was a testament to the evolving nature of my healing process, a continuous journey of experimentation and refinement.

One of my favorite combinations became a vibrant blend of apples, carrots, ginger, celery, and turmeric. The sweetness of the carrots balanced the spicy kick of the ginger, while the tanginess of the orange added a refreshing counterpoint. This juice became a potent ally in combating inflammation, boosting my immunity, and invigorating my system. This concoction was a nutritional powerhouse, brimming with antioxidants and vitamins that nourished my cells and enhanced my overall well-being.

My kitchen used to be a space of culinary struggle, but now it is a vibrant hub of healthy creation. The juicer became a central fixture, a symbol of my dedication to my health. The rhythmic whirring of the machine, the vibrant colors of the fruits and vegetables, and the satisfying clink of the glass as I poured the freshly squeezed juice—these all became integral elements of my morning ritual, transforming a simple act of nourishment into a meditation on self-care.

As the weeks turned into months, I began to notice significant changes in my body. My digestion improved, my inflammation decreased, and my energy levels soared. My skin became clearer, my sleep more restful, and my overall sense of well-being increased. These changes weren't immediate; they were gradual, subtle improvements that accumulated over time, reinforcing my commitment to this lifestyle change.

If you're reading this feeling disconnected from your body—tired, inflamed, sick, or stuck—I want you to know I see you. I was you. And I promise you this: You can start again. One small shift at a time.

The Wake-Up Call I Didn't Want, But Needed

I'll never forget the moment I broke down at the hospital. Lying in that bed, hooked to machines, swollen from the inside out, I asked myself a question that changed my life:

"What if I could love myself enough to take care of this body I've been fighting for so long?"

That question became my turning point.

I didn't need another diet. I needed a reset. A rebirth. A new relationship with the body I lived in. I realized that food wasn't the enemy, but neither was my body. I had spent years punishing it, criticizing it, pushing it, ignoring its needs.

It was time to listen. To nurture. To heal.

Food as Fuel, Not Fix

I started simple. I didn't do anything drastic. I just asked myself each day:

"Will this fuel my healing or feed my pain?"

One of the most significant shifts came when I began drinking celery juice every morning. It wasn't magic, but it was medicine for me. It felt clean. It reduced inflammation. It gave my gut a break. More than anything, it symbolized intentionality; that I was choosing to care for myself on purpose.

From there, I began reducing processed foods, sugar, and anything that left me feeling heavy, bloated, or drained. I didn't restrict. I replaced. I added more greens, anti-inflammatory foods, water, teas, and things that felt alive.

But I also fed myself emotionally, taking breaks, eating in peace, blessing my meals, slowing down enough to chew, taste, and be present with my food.

Fueling your body isn't just about what's on your plate. It's about how you eat, when you eat, why you eat, and who you become when you're eating from a place of worth.

What Are You Really Feeding Yourself?

Take a moment to think about this: What are you feeding yourself every single day?

- Physically (food, drink, medication, supplements)
- Mentally (thoughts, beliefs, stories, self-talk)
- Emotionally (stress, joy, guilt, shame)
- Spiritually (faith, hope, connection, stillness)

It all matters.

If you're eating greens but drowning in stress, your body still feels unsafe. If you're drinking water but feeding yourself fear all day, you're still inflamed. This is why fueling your body must be holistic, because you are a holistic being.

This isn't about rules. It's about relationships. Not just what you put in your mouth, but what you say to yourself after.

I used to eat something and immediately criticize myself.

"You shouldn't have had that."

"No wonder you're bloated."

"Why can't you just eat clean like other women?"

No food nourishes a body that feels judged.

So I stopped shaming myself. And I started choosing love.

Blueprint Steps: Fuel Your Body with Intention

Here's your Unshakable blueprint for fueling your body:

1. Ask yourself before each meal: Will this bring me closer to healing or further from it?

   This simple pause creates mindful eating. Start paying attention to how you feel before, during, and after meals—not just what you eat.

2. Begin your day with something pure.

   Whether it's celery juice, lemon water, or a prayer of gratitude before your first bite—let your morning ritual be an act of nourishment.

3. Crowd out inflammation with nourishment.

   Instead of focusing on restriction, ADD more healing foods: leafy greens, berries, omega-rich fats, clean protein, and anti-inflammatory teas. The more goodness you bring in, the less room there is for what harms.

4. Heal your relationship with food.

   No more guilt, shame, or self-sabotage. Food is not the enemy. Begin blessing your meals, slowing down, and thanking your body for what it can digest, absorb, and heal.

5. Fuel your life, not just your body.

   What music are you listening to? What shows are you watching? What energy are you absorbing online?

Be just as selective with your mental diet as you are with your physical one.

- You can't heal a body you criticize every time you eat.

- Your body is not the enemy—it's the messenger.
- Every bite either fights inflammation or feeds it.
- You don't need to eat perfectly. You need to eat lovingly.
- The most powerful detox is self-respect.

What I Eat Isn't What Heals Me—It's the Way I Honor Myself

My healing didn't come from a perfect meal plan or some magical green smoothie. It came from changing the way I saw myself. I began fueling my body because I believed I was worth taking care of.

That's the difference.

You can drink all the green juice in the world, but if you're swallowing it with shame or rushing through it like a task to check off, your nervous system still feels threatened. It's not about what you do—it's about how you do it.

I fuel my body from a place of compassion now. I listen to it. I bless it. I thank it. I don't punish it for being in pain—I honor it for showing up anyway.

Journal Prompt: Fueling From Love

Take time to reflect and write:

1. What's one small change I can make this week to fuel my body with love and intention?
2. How do I want to feel after I eat?
3. What has my relationship with food been like, and how can I shift it toward kindness and healing?
4. What is one small shift I can make today to show my body more love through nourishment? Think simple: a glass of water, a whole-food snack, a slower pace at lunch.
5. What would it feel like to honor my body instead of fighting it?

Describe in detail what a day of nourishment, intention, and grace could look like.

_____

_____

_____

_____

_____

_____

_____

_____

_____

You Are Worth Nourishment

No matter what your past has looked like, and no matter how disconnected you may feel right now…

You are not too far gone. You are not too late.

You are allowed to start again.

Start by adding one thing that brings your body peace.

Start by letting go of one habit that leaves you inflamed.

Start by listening—not judging.

Fueling your body is an act of love.

And love is the most powerful medicine of all.

You're not doing this to lose weight, to impress anyone, or to follow a trend.

You're doing it because you are worthy of feeling vibrant, clear, alive, and aligned.

You are worthy of nourishment.

You are worthy of feeling good in your body again.

You are worthy of being fully well.

And it all begins here.

Bridging Into Mindset: From Fuel to Foundation

Fueling your body isn't just about the food.

It's about the story behind the food. The reason you choose to care or the reason you don't.

It's about the beliefs that shape your choices and the inner dialogue you carry while trying to heal.

And that brings us to something deeper—your mindset.

Because no matter how well you eat, how many supplements you take, or how many routines you follow, if your mind is full of fear, guilt, shame, or old limiting beliefs, your body will still feel unsafe.

"Your mindset is the soil where every habit grows."

If the soil is toxic, the seeds won't bloom.

But if the soil is healthy—full of belief, truth, and love—everything begins to shift.

In Chapter 5, we'll go deeper into how I began to change not just what I did, but how I thought.

How I rewrote the story in my head.

How I stopped letting fear run the show.

And how I began speaking to myself like someone I loved.

Because if food is the fuel...

Mindset is the ignition.

And together, they'll carry you toward the unshakable life you were born to live.

Pillar 2 – Master Your Mindset

I used to believe my body was the enemy.

I blamed it for everything: my pain, my exhaustion, my limitations.

And behind that blame was a narrative I didn't even realize I was telling myself.

"You're not strong enough."

"You'll always be sick."

"You're falling behind."

"You're not doing enough."

"You're not enough."

It wasn't until I began doing the deeper inner work that I realized:

My body wasn't the problem; my mindset was.

Because even as I started fueling my body with intention, something was still missing.

I had changed my habits... but I hadn't changed my headspace.

I was still thinking like the sick version of me.

Still waiting for someone to give me permission to believe I could get better.

Still waking up each day expecting the worst.

And nothing outside of me would shift until something inside me did.

That shift began the day I put pen to paper.

Journaling: Rewriting My Story Through the Mirror of Truth

There was a time I felt completely disconnected from the woman I used to be. I looked in the mirror and didn't recognize her. I was exhausted, in pain, and overwhelmed. My body hurt, my mind raced, and my heart carried a weight I couldn't name.

Living with chronic illness had stripped away so many pieces of my identity that I didn't know where to begin rebuilding. But what helped me start wasn't a big, dramatic breakthrough. It was something small—something simple. A pen. A notebook. And five quiet minutes with myself.

Journaling saved my mindset.

That might sound dramatic, but I mean it. Journaling became my lifeline when everything felt too loud, too overwhelming, too painful. It gave me space to breathe and permission to release the fears I had buried deep. And it helped me create a new story when the old one had nearly broken me.

The practice became a crucial component of my self-discovery. The pages were filled with a record of my physical and emotional experiences, providing a valuable tool for identifying patterns, recognizing progress, and charting my path toward healing. It became a record of my struggles, my victories, and the gradual shift in my perspective from victimhood to empowerment.

At first, I didn't know what to write.

So I started with what I felt.

"I'm scared. I'm exhausted. I don't want to live like this anymore."

There it was, raw, real, messy truth.

And something about writing it made me feel lighter.

Like I was finally being heard, even if it was just by the page.

Over time, I stopped just releasing pain and started rewriting possibility.

I wrote about the woman I wanted to become.

I wrote letters to the future version of me.

I wrote prayers, mantras, hopes, and visions.

I released guilt.

I forgave myself.

I told the truth, then I told a better one.

I started with something I could handle, **gratitude.**

I didn't think I had anything to be grateful for at first.

How could I, when I was living in pain and barely functioning?

However, I kept hearing that gratitude could change everything.

So, I gave it a try.

Every morning, I wrote down three things I was grateful for.

Some days, it was easy. I'd write:

- "Warm tea."
- "Birdsong outside."
- "My daughters giving me a hug."

Some days it was small:

- "My daughters' laughter."
- "A hot cup of coffee."
- "A walk in the sunshine."

But other days, especially when I felt heavy with pain or fear, I remember digging deep and writing:

- "I'm grateful I got out of bed."
- "I'm grateful I didn't give up."
- "I'm grateful I still believe healing is possible."

It wasn't just about finding the good. It was about training my brain to look for it.

Gratitude journaling began to rewire my perspective on the world. Instead of focusing on what I had lost—my energy, my strength, my old life—I began to see what I still had: breath, love, resilience, and the power to choose again. That shift wasn't overnight, but it was powerful. Gratitude softened the edges of my suffering and gave me access to joy, even on the hard days.

But I didn't stop at gratitude. Soon, I started writing about my pain, my thoughts, and the stories I was telling myself. And wow—those stories were heavy.

I realized how often I was speaking to myself in a way I'd never speak to someone I loved. My journal became a mirror. I saw the lies I had been repeating for years: "You're not enough. You're failing. You're a burden. You'll never get better."

No wonder I was stuck.

That's when something shifted. I decided to stop writing about my pain and start writing through it. I began to rewrite the narrative. I challenged those thoughts. When the voice said, "You'll never heal," I wrote back: "I am healing, even if it doesn't look the way I imagined." When the voice said, "You're too broken," I responded: "I'm not broken—I'm becoming."

This wasn't toxic positivity. It was deep self-respect. It was truth-telling. It was refusing to let the illness define who I was or where I was going.

My journal became the place where I reclaimed my voice.

One day, I wrote a letter to the girl I used to be. Another day, I wrote a letter to the woman I was becoming. Both made me cry. But both helped me forgive the past and believe in the future. Writing those words down helped me shift from "Why is this happening to me?" to "What is this here to teach me?"

What I didn't expect was how fast it shifted me.

Not because my pain vanished, but because my perspective did.

Gratitude rewired my brain to look for good.

To find light in the dark.

To speak life when fear tried to take over.

It softened me.

It reminded me that even on hard days, there's still beauty to be found.

After all this realization in my journaling, visualization came into the picture.

Visualization: Becoming Who I Was Meant to Be

Each morning, after journaling my gratitude and rewriting my thoughts, I'd close my eyes and imagine a version of myself who felt vibrant, energized, and joyful. I'd picture her walking on the beach, laughing with her girls, speaking on a stage, glowing from the inside out.

She didn't just look different—she felt different.

She felt light. Unburdened. Unshakable.

At first, she felt like a dream. But the more I visualized her, the more real she became.

Over time, that version of me stopped being a fantasy and began to become my blueprint.

I started visualizing the version of me I wanted to become.

Not the "perfect" version. Not the "pain-free" version.

But the empowered version.

I would close my eyes and see her:

Walking with ease.

Laughing with joy.

Living without fear.

Moving through her day with calm, purpose, and radiance.

I'd feel her energy. I'd see her life. I'd become her in my mind.

And the more I did it, the more I started living into her.

Visualization became a practice of embodiment—of acting now like the woman I was becoming.

Not waiting until I was "better" to feel whole.

Not waiting until I looked healed to believe I was.

It was training my brain to expect good.

And the brain, as science shows us, begins to believe what you show it consistently.

Visualization is powerful because it gives your brain a roadmap. It helps you align your thoughts, energy, and choices with the future you want to create. It taught me to make decisions not based on where I was, but where I was going.

I asked myself: "What would the healthy, happy version of me do today?" Sometimes the answer was "Rest." Other times, it was "Move your body. Speak kindly. Choose joy." That daily practice of imagining a better version of myself gave me the strength to become her.

Rewriting My Story: From Victim to Victor

I had to get honest about the stories I was telling myself every day.

Stories like:

- "My illness controls me."
- "I'll never get my life back."

- "I'm falling behind."

Those stories were shaping how I felt, how I moved, and how I showed up.

They were keeping me small. Stuck. Silent.

So I started rewriting them.

I wrote:

- "My body is not broken—it's wise."
- "I am learning how to heal in a way that honors me."
- "I'm not behind—I'm becoming."

I spoke these new truths out loud.

I wrote them again and again.

And slowly, my story changed—not because my circumstances did, but because **I** did.

Affirmations: Speaking Life Over Myself

If I could tell you one tool that helped me the most—it's this: affirmations.

Not cheesy ones. Not fluff. Not fake positivity.

Real, soul-grounding, life-giving affirmations.

I wrote them. I spoke them. I recorded them. I stuck them on mirrors, dashboards, and journals.

Because the way we talk to ourselves matters.

Your brain believes in repetition.

And if all it ever hears is "you're not enough," it will believe that.

But if you start saying:

- "I am worthy."
- "I am healing."
- "I am more than my pain."
- "I am enough, even when I feel undone."

Something powerful happens.

You begin to rise.

The biggest transformation of my life didn't happen because of what I did.

It happened because of how I thought.

For years, I let my mindset keep me stuck.

- I told myself, I'm always going to feel like this.
- I believed, My body was broken. There's nothing I can do.
- I assumed, This is just my life now. There's no point in hoping for more.

And because I thought those things?

I lived as if they were true.

Until the day I learned one simple truth that changed everything:

Your thoughts shape your reality.

Not in some fluffy, "just think positive" way.

But in a scientific, undeniable way.

Because the way you think about yourself, your health, and your future determines the choices you make.

And those choices?

They shape your entire life.

The Invisible Battle: How Your Mindset Controls Your Life

For years, I didn't realize I was in a battle.

Not with my body.

Not with my diagnosis.

Not with my circumstances.

But with my own mind.

Every single day, we have thousands of thoughts.

Most of them?

They're the same thoughts we had yesterday.

And if you've been living in fear, doubt, or frustration for years, your brain has been reinforcing those thoughts over and over.

Until they become your beliefs.

And once something becomes a belief, your brain does everything it can to prove it right.

That's why when I believed:

"I'll never get better." → I saw proof everywhere.

"This is just how life is now." → I stopped looking for solutions.

"I'm stuck." → I made choices that kept me stuck.

I wasn't stuck because of my illness.

I was stuck because of my mindset.

And if I wanted to change my life?

I had to change the way I thought about it first.

What Story Are You Telling Yourself?

I want you to think about this for a moment:

What are you telling yourself every single day?

Because whether you realize it or not—

You have a story running in your mind.

And that story?

It's shaping your life.

Are you telling yourself:

- I'm healing, little by little.
- I am capable of figuring this out.
- There is hope for me.

Or are you telling yourself:

- I'll never get better.
- I'm stuck, and nothing will change.
- Why even try? It's not worth it.

Because here's the truth:

Your brain will find proof for whatever you believe.

If you believe you're stuck? You'll see reasons why you're stuck.

If you believe healing is possible? You'll find ways to make it possible.

So let me ask you—

What story have you been telling yourself?

And more importantly—

Is it time to change it?

Rewiring Your Brain for Healing & Growth

Once I realized how powerful my thoughts were, I made a decision.

I wasn't going to let my old beliefs control me anymore.

I was going to rewire my brain.

And here's how I did it:

1. I Became Aware of My Thoughts

At first, I didn't even realize how negative my thinking was.

So, I started paying attention.

Every time I had a thought like, "This is too hard," or "I'll never feel better," I caught it.

I didn't judge myself.

I just noticed.

Because you can't change what you don't recognize.

2. I Challenged My Old Beliefs

Once I became aware of my thoughts, I started questioning them.

Was it really true that I'd never feel better?

Had I really tried everything to improve my health?

Was I really stuck—or was that just what I had convinced myself?

Most of the time?

My thoughts weren't facts.

They were just old stories I had repeated for years.

And stories?

Can be rewritten.

3. I Replaced the Negative Thoughts with New Ones

Every time I caught myself thinking something negative, I didn't just stop the thought.

I replaced it.

Instead of: I'm stuck. → I told myself: I am figuring this out, one step at a time.

Instead of: I'll always feel this way. → I told myself: My body is capable of healing in small ways.

Instead of: This is impossible. → I told myself: I am learning what works for me.

At first, it felt fake.

Like I was lying to myself.

But over time?

It became my new truth.

And my actions followed.

I stopped feeling defeated.

I started looking for solutions.

I took my power back.

Because when you change your thoughts?

You change your choices.

And when you change your choices?

You change your life.

Healing Tools to Take Back Your Power

Journaling, gratitude, and visualization—they weren't just habits. They were healing tools. They helped me take back my power. They gave me a safe space to process, reflect, and create a new future one page at a time.

This practice didn't cost anything. I didn't need a perfect morning routine or the perfect notebook. I just needed to show up. To be honest, to be gentle, and to be willing to believe that something could change.

And it did.

The more I practiced gratitude, the more joy I found.

The more I rewrote my thoughts, the more empowered I felt.

The more I visualized healing, the more aligned my life became.

These tools helped me rebuild my mindset from the inside out. They helped me stop living from fear and start living from faith. They helped me stop surviving and start creating.

If you're reading this and you feel overwhelmed by the noise in your mind, the weight of your past, or the pain in your present, start small.

Grab a pen. Write three things you're grateful for.

Speak kindly to yourself in writing.

Imagine who you want to become.

Do it again tomorrow. And the next day. Let the words become a bridge between where you are and where you're going.

You don't have to be perfect. You just have to be willing.

Your journal doesn't judge you. It doesn't expect anything from you. It simply holds space. And sometimes, space is exactly what you need to breathe, to process, and to rise again.

You are not your diagnosis. You are not your pain. You are not the story you were told. You get to write a new one.

One page at a time.

Learning to Live and Thrive in the Present

Thriving in the present doesn't mean ignoring your pain or forgetting all that you've been through – it means creating space for stillness, awareness, and gentle growth in the middle of chaos.

One particularly effective technique was mindful breathing.

Simply focusing on the rhythm of my breath—the inhale and exhale—provided a grounding presence, a gentle anchor that pulled me back to the present whenever my mind wandered into the spiral of worries and anxieties about the future or regrets about the past.

This practice could be done anywhere, anytime: during a yoga session, while waiting for an appointment, or even in the middle of a stressful day. The simplicity of the breathing technique was exactly what made it so powerful. It helped me feel centered and focused when I needed it most.

Another crucial element of embracing the present moment was cultivating gratitude. I began to actively seek out and appreciate the small joys in life, the things that were easily overlooked in my previous state of constant striving. The kindness of a friend, the beauty of a sunset, the comfort of a warm blanket—these seemingly trivial occurrences became sources of immense contentment when viewed through the lens of gratitude. I started journaling regularly, documenting these moments of appreciation, creating a tangible record of the good in my life that helped to counterbalance the negativity associated with my chronic illness.

This practice of gratitude extended beyond simple daily observations. I found that expressing appreciation to others—whether through a heartfelt thank-you note, a simple compliment, or a thoughtful gesture—not only brought joy to the recipient but also deepened my own sense of well-being. The act of giving, of acknowledging the positive contributions of others, fostered a sense of connection and purpose that rose above the limitations of my physical condition.

Mindfulness wasn't about ignoring the challenges or pretending that everything was perfect. Rather, it was about acknowledging both the joys and the struggles, accepting them as real parts of the present moment without judgment. This involved learning to observe my thoughts and emotions without getting swept away by them, recognizing that thoughts and feelings are temporary, like clouds passing across the sky.

This journey of acceptance involved confronting my fear of the future, a fear that had been a constant companion for years. I learned to reframe my perspective, viewing my challenges not as impossible obstacles but as opportunities for growth and learning. This shift in perspective was not always easy, often requiring conscious effort and self-compassion. There were setbacks and moments of intense frustration, times when the weight of chronic illness seemed overwhelming. But through perseverance and consistent mindfulness practice, I developed the strength to navigate these moments with greater calm and resilience.

Learning to show myself compassion became an indispensable tool in my journey. This meant treating myself with the same kindness and understanding that I would offer a dear friend struggling with similar challenges. It involved letting go of self-criticism and replacing it with self-acceptance, recognizing that I was doing the best I could given my circumstances. This wasn't about complacency; it was about honoring my limitations without giving in to negative thoughts or self-talk..

One of the most significant benefits of embracing the present moment was the enhanced appreciation for human connection. By actively engaging in mindful interactions with others, truly listening to their stories, and sharing my own experiences authentically, I deepened my relationships and forged new connections. This appreciation for human connection extended beyond personal interactions. I found a sense of belonging and support in online communities dedicated to chronic illness, where we shared experiences and offered encouragement to others navigating similar journeys.

Furthermore, mindfulness helped me to develop a greater appreciation for the beauty that surrounded me, even in the most mundane aspects of life. A simple flower in a crack in the sidewalk, the way sunlight filtered through the leaves on a tree, the laughter of children at play—these moments, previously unnoticed, became sources of wonder and joy. This deepened sense of appreciation made everyday existence more vibrant and meaningful.

My practice of mindfulness wasn't limited to specific times or places. It became integrated into the fabric of my daily life, influencing my interactions with others, my approach to challenges, and my overall perspective. It wasn't a quick fix or a magic solution, but a continuous process of learning, growing, and evolving.

The transformation wasn't immediate or effortless; it involved persistent effort and a willingness to adapt my practices as needed. There were days when mindfulness felt elusive, when my mind raced with anxieties, and the present moment felt overwhelming. But even on those days, the simple act of returning to my breath, even for a few seconds, provided a moment of calm, a brief anchor in the storm. Over time, these small moments of grounding accumulated, leading to a more sustained sense of presence and peace.

Through persistent practice, the present moment became less a fleeting destination and more a continuous state of being. This state of being, in turn, allowed me to find joy and fulfillment even amidst the challenges of chronic illness, transforming my relationship with suffering and empowering me to live a life not merely of survival, but of profound and authentic thriving. The journey of embracing the present moment is ongoing, a continuous process of refinement and adaptation, but the rewards are immeasurable. It's a journey of continuous self-discovery, a life lived fully and authentically, in every breath and every moment.

The Key to True Transformation

Here's what I want you to know:

The way you think about yourself, your health, and your future determines everything.

It's not just about positive thinking.

It's about training your brain to work for you, not against you.

Because your brain?

It's listening.

To every word you say.

To every belief you hold.

To every thought you repeat.

And when you change those thoughts?

You change your reality.

Because remember: your brain believes what you tell it.

So, tell it a story worth believing.

Now that we've rewritten the story in our minds, we need to address something else: the things we're still holding onto.

Because true transformation?

It's not just about adding new habits.

It's about letting go of what no longer serves you.

Journal Prompt: Rewriting Your Story

Take a moment to reflect. Grab a journal and answer these questions honestly:

1. What is one negative thought you've been telling yourself for years?
2. Where did that belief come from? Is it actually true?
3. What is a new belief you can choose to replace it with?
4. How will your life change if you start thinking this way?

Blueprint Steps: Master Your Mindset

Here is your Unshakable blueprint to transform your mindset from the inside out:

1. Start a daily journaling practice.

Write what you feel. Release it. Then write what you want to believe. Use prompts like:

- "What do I need to let go of today?"
- "What truth do I want to live by?"

2. Practice 3 daily gratitudes.

Write them every morning or night. Look for the little things—they will lead you to the big things.

3. Visualize the woman you're becoming.

Close your eyes. Picture her in vivid detail. Step into her mindset. Ask: How would she show up today?

4. Rewrite one old belief each week.

Take a limiting belief you've been carrying and reframe it into truth. Speak it. Write it. Live it.

5. Say your affirmations out loud.

Start with these:

- "I am enough."
- "I am healing."
- "I choose peace."
- "I am unshakable."

Remember:

- You can't heal a life built on thoughts that keep you stuck.
- Your story doesn't end where pain began.
- Every new thought is a step toward freedom.
- Speak life over yourself like your healing depends on it—because it does.
- What you believe about yourself becomes the world you live in. Choose wisely.

6. Live and thrive in the present moment by applying mindset mastery practices like mindful breathing, practicing gratitude, and reclaiming your self-compassion in your day-to-day life.

From Thought to Movement

Once I began to master my mindset, something beautiful happened: I wanted to move again.

Not because I was trying to lose weight.

Not because I "had to."

But because I felt inspired. Alive. Grateful.

And that's where we go next.

Because the most powerful movement isn't driven by shame—it's driven by love.

When your mindset aligns with healing, your body naturally follows.

And the way you move becomes a reflection of how deeply you've come home to yourself.

CHAPTER 6

Pillar 3 – Move Your Body with Love

For a long time, I believed movement had to be intense to be effective.

I thought if I wasn't sweating, pushing through pain, or completely worn out after a workout... it didn't count.

I punished my body with movement. I didn't move because I loved her; I moved because I was trying to fix her.

Exercise used to feel like punishment.

If I wasn't exhausted, drenched in sweat, or pushing through pain, I didn't think it counted.

But my body needed nourishment, not punishment.

I started moving in ways that felt good:

- Daily walks in nature (Sunlight, fresh air, grounding myself)
- Gentle stretching & yoga (Building strength without inflaming my joints)
- Restorative movement (Learning to listen to what my body actually needed)

My first attempts at increasing my movement were humbling. The simplest tasks, things most people take for granted, felt monumental. Walking to the mailbox, a distance of perhaps fifty feet, left me breathless and aching. The stairs leading to my bedroom became a daily Everest, each step a victory hard-won. The chronic pain, a familiar companion, flared up with increased intensity after even the slightest exertion. Fatigue, that persistent shadow that had clung to me for years, intensified, leaving me slumped on the sofa, depleted and discouraged.

The initial lack of motivation was perhaps the greatest hurdle. The years of inactivity, dictated by pain and exhaustion, had instilled a sense of helplessness. The idea of embarking on a program of physical activity felt overwhelming, an impossible mountain I wasn't sure I could even begin to climb. My mind imagined images of painful workouts, strenuous exercises, and eventual failure, reinforcing the negative self-talk that had become so ingrained. I found myself making excuses, procrastinating, and finding reasons to avoid any physical exertion. The comfort of staying still was a powerful pull, tempting me back to the familiar limitations of a life where movement was minimal. Overcoming this mental barrier proved more challenging than the physical limitations themselves.

But I knew, deep down, that remaining inactive wasn't an option. My physical and emotional well-being depended on breaking free from this cycle of pain and immobility. I realized that I didn't need to run a marathon or lift weights to achieve progress. My journey towards increased mobility would be a marathon, not a sprint, a gradual progression of small, incremental steps. I started by setting realistic goals, focusing on achievable targets rather than aiming for ambitious feats that were likely to lead to discouragement.

My first step involved simply walking around my living room. I started with five minutes, a seemingly insignificant amount of time, but enough to challenge my limited stamina. I concentrated on maintaining an upright posture to alleviate strain on my back and hips. I focused on my breathing, slowing it down to promote relaxation and minimize discomfort. I paid close attention to my body's signals, stopping whenever I felt any sharp pain or overwhelming fatigue. These initial sessions were less about physical exertion and more about cultivating a mindful awareness of my body's capabilities and limitations.

As my tolerance improved, I gradually increased the duration of my living room walks. Ten minutes, then fifteen, then twenty. I started incorporating simple stretches and gentle movements that eased stiffness and improved flexibility. I focused on range-of-motion exercises, slowly extending my limbs, feeling the muscles stretch and release. The initial stiffness gradually eased, giving way to a growing sense of suppleness and flexibility. My body felt less like a rigid, aching cage and more like a capable, responsive part of me, finally listening to my gentle guidance.

Once I felt comfortable walking in my living room, I moved my exercise regimen to my backyard. Initially, this was a short walk around my patio, again focusing on my posture, my breathing, and my body's signals. Gradually, I expanded my routine, stepping onto the grass, feeling the cool earth beneath my feet. The change of scenery provided a welcome distraction from the repetitive nature of indoor exercise, helping me overcome the boredom that sometimes threatened to derail my progress.

Over time, the short strolls around my backyard became longer walks along the quiet streets of my neighborhood. I started with a short block, monitoring my body's response, then two blocks, then three. These walks were a powerful experience. Not only were they improving my physical condition, but they were also opening up a whole new world of sensory experiences. The sights, sounds, and smells of my neighborhood, which had once been overlooked in my previous state of confinement, filled me with a sense of awe and gratitude.

The people in my neighborhood became part of my recovery journey. The friendly greetings, the shared smiles, and the simple acts of human connection provided a much-needed boost to my morale. These small interactions became a crucial element of my healing process, reminding me that I wasn't alone in my struggle and that a supportive community was surrounding me.

I began to incorporate walking into my daily routine. Instead of driving to the local grocery store, I started walking, carrying a small basket for my groceries. This was initially a challenging task, but with each trip, I found myself gaining strength and stamina. The sense of accomplishment that accompanied these daily walks was immense. It wasn't just about the physical exercise; it was about reclaiming my independence, my ability to move freely and participate fully in my life.

My increased mobility also expanded my horizons beyond my immediate surroundings. I started exploring the nearby parks, enjoying the fresh air, the sunlight, and the beauty of the natural world. Initially, my excursions were limited to short, gentle strolls, but as my fitness improved, I gradually increased the distance and intensity of my walks. These outings became a source of immense joy and rejuvenation, filling me with a sense of wonder and gratitude.

The journey wasn't without its setbacks. There were days when the pain flared up, days when fatigue overwhelmed me, days when the temptation to give up was almost too strong to resist. However, I learned to recognize these setbacks as temporary obstacles, not impossible barriers. I adapted my exercise regimen to accommodate my fluctuating energy levels, focusing on rest and recovery when needed.

I discovered the importance of listening to my body, of paying attention to its signals, and respecting its limits. I learned to differentiate between the discomfort of exertion and the sharp pain of injury. I adjusted my pace, modified my movements, and embraced rest as an essential component of my recovery process. This mindful approach helped me avoid injuries and maintain my momentum.

One of the most unexpected benefits of increased mobility was the improvement in my mental state. The regular exercise helped alleviate stress, reduce anxiety, and boost my mood. The physical activity released endorphins, those natural mood elevators, leaving me feeling invigorated and optimistic. The increased exposure to sunlight also helped regulate my sleep patterns, improving my overall quality of sleep.

The improved sleep, in turn, fueled my physical recovery, creating a positive feedback loop that propelled my progress forward. The reduction in fatigue allowed me to engage in more physical activity, which in turn reduced stress and improved sleep, further strengthening my physical and mental resilience. This positive cycle became the cornerstone of my healing process.

My journey towards reclaiming my body wasn't about achieving some idealized level of fitness; it was about gradually restoring my mobility, my independence, and my sense of self. It was about learning to listen to my body, honoring its limits, and celebrating every small victory along the way. It was about finding joy in movement, not just as a means to an end but as a way of experiencing life to the fullest. The journey continues, a lifelong commitment to nurturing my body and mind, one step at a time.

My newfound ability to walk, even short distances, opened up a world of possibilities. It wasn't just about the physical act of putting one foot in front of the other; it was about reconnecting with my surroundings, experiencing the world through my senses once more. The initially simple walks around my neighborhood became increasingly enriching. I began to notice the beauty in the everyday-the bright bursts of flowers in bloom, the deep greens of palm-lined paths, and the gentle sway of summer branches in the breeze. The familiar streets took on a new vibrancy, each walk revealing details I had previously missed during my years of confinement.

The sights weren't the only things that captivated me. The sounds of the neighborhood – the chirping of birds, the distant hum of traffic, the laughter of children at play – became a soothing symphony. I rediscovered the simple pleasures of hearing the world around me, the richness of sounds I had grown accustomed to filtering out. Even the smells – the fragrance of freshly cut grass, the earthy scent of rain-soaked soil, or the sweet aroma of blossoms in the spring – filled my senses with a sense of renewal and wonder. These sensory experiences were profoundly restorative, a balm for the soul, revitalizing my spirit in ways I never anticipated.

Gradually, my walks grew longer and more ambitious. I began exploring the local parks, finding solace in the serenity of nature. The parks offered a diverse range of landscapes: paved paths for gentler strolls, winding trails for more challenging walks, and open spaces for leisurely strolls. The rhythmic movement of walking became meditative, a form of moving meditation, that cleared my mind and freed my thoughts. I began to appreciate the simple act of breathing deeply, filling my lungs with fresh air, and feeling the energy of the earth beneath my feet.

The parks weren't just places for physical exercise; they became sanctuaries, spaces for introspection and self-discovery. I found myself observing the intricate details of nature – the delicate patterns on a butterfly's wings, the finely woven web of a spider, the vibrant colors of a wildflower. These small details, often overlooked in the hustle and bustle of daily life, filled me with a sense of awe and appreciation for the beauty of the natural world. The quiet solitude of the parks was an undeniable contrast to the noise and demands of daily living. It provided the space for reflection, allowing me to process my thoughts and emotions and ultimately find a deeper sense of peace and contentment.

My walking routine became a source of both physical and emotional well-being. The increased mobility led to improved cardiovascular fitness, increased energy levels, and a stronger sense of trust in my body and my own capabilities. But it was the emotional benefits that surprised me the most. The simple act of walking became a way to reduce stress, to clear my head, and to connect with the natural world around me.

Walking, however, wasn't the only form of movement I embraced. I had always been intrigued by yoga, its emphasis on mindful movement and breath control. Initially, I approached yoga with apprehension, fearing that the flexibility and strength required would be beyond my capabilities. However, I discovered that there were various styles of yoga, each with its own emphasis and intensity. I began with gentle, restorative yoga, focusing on poses that promoted relaxation and improved flexibility.

I found a local studio that offered beginner classes and a supportive and welcoming environment. The instructors were patient and understanding, adapting the poses to suit individual needs and limitations. They encouraged a mindful approach to the practice, emphasizing the importance of listening to one's body and respecting its limitations. I learned to nurture a greater awareness of my body, noticing the subtle sensations in my muscles and joints. The focus on breath control helped me to relax and to release tension, both physically and mentally.

Movement, once a daunting task, became a source of empowerment. I started with short walks in my garden, gradually increasing the duration and intensity as my strength allowed. I incorporated gentle chair yoga and stretching exercises into my daily routine. These small acts of self-care became moments of mindful connection with my body, rituals that nurtured both my physical and mental well-being. The physical improvements were noticeable, but the mental and emotional benefits were transformational. The act of exercising choice over my physical activity was deeply empowering.

And instead of hating my body for its limitations, I began to thank it for what it could do.

But when my body broke down, when I found myself unable to lift my head off the pillow without pain or fatigue, I had to face a truth I'd been running from:

My body wasn't failing me. She was protecting me.

And I had ignored her for far too long.

That was the beginning of a completely different relationship with movement—one rooted in love, not punishment. In compassion, not control. In rest, not rigidity.

It took getting sick, slowing down, and learning how trauma and stress live in the body for me to understand this:

The body keeps the score. And movement is how we begin to rewrite the story.

My Wake-Up Call: Redefining What Movement Means

When I was at my sickest, I could barely walk across the room. My muscles ached. My joints screamed. My nervous system was so fried I couldn't tolerate even the smallest effort.

The girl who used to run and lift weights was gone—and I grieved her.

But in that stillness, something else emerged.

A softness. A presence. A curiosity.

One day, I stood outside and walked for five minutes—no timer, no goal. Just me and the wind, my feet on the earth, and my breath.

I cried. Not because it hurt. But because, for the first time, it felt like love.

That's when I knew I didn't need to move harder—I needed to move kinder.

And in that moment, I gave myself permission to start over.

The Body Remembers What the Mind Tries to Forget

Books like The Body Keeps the Score: Brain, Mind, and Body in the Healing of Trauma by Bessel van der Kolk opened my eyes to what my own body had been trying to tell me.

The pain I carried wasn't just physical.

It was emotional. Layered. Stored in places I hadn't touched in years.

The fear of never being good enough.

The guilt for slowing down.

The grief of losing who I used to be.

It turns out that when we don't process stress, trauma, or emotion, it doesn't disappear.

Stored in muscles. In breath. In posture. In tension. In fatigue.

And the longer we hold it in, the heavier we become.

When My Body Spoke, I Finally Listened

I spent years trying to fix my body—chasing treatments, adjusting my diet, and searching for anything that could give me relief.

- My joints ached, my muscles throbbed, and exhaustion became my constant companion.
- I was diagnosed with Rheumatoid Arthritis and Fibromyalgia, and doctors told me that my body was attacking itself.
- No matter what I did, the pain and inflammation never fully went away.

For the longest time, I believed this was purely a physical problem—that my body was simply breaking down. But what I didn't realize was that my body wasn't just reacting to food or medications—it was responding to my emotions, my past traumas, and my stress.

- When I was overwhelmed, my symptoms worsened.
- When I held onto resentment, my body tightened with pain.
- When I felt emotionally exhausted, my energy was completely drained.

And the moment I started to address not just my physical health, but my emotional and mental well-being?

That was when my healing truly began.

Because what I learned—what changed everything—was this: your body keeps score of everything you've been through.

Every unprocessed emotion.

Every unresolved trauma.

Every moment of stress you've suppressed instead of expressed.

And if you don't deal with what's happening internally?

Your body will carry it for you.

The Truth About Trauma, Stress & Your Body

Most people think trauma is something that only affects your mind.

But the truth?

Your body remembers everything.

The stress you never dealt with.

The emotions you never processed.

The moments you pushed through instead of honoring what you needed.

And over time, that emotional burden can show up as:

- Chronic pain
- Inflammation
- Digestive issues
- Autoimmune disorders
- Fatigue
- Anxiety and depression

Because your nervous system doesn't know the difference between past pain and present pain.

If trauma, grief, or stress were never properly processed, your body remains stuck in survival mode, believing it is still under attack.

Your muscles tighten.

Your immune system goes into overdrive.

Your body stays inflamed and exhausted—because it doesn't know it's safe.

This is why healing isn't just about managing symptoms.

It's about addressing the root cause—the stress, emotions, and unprocessed trauma that have been weighing you down.

How Is Your Body Holding On?

I want you to take a moment and ask yourself—

Where is my body holding onto stress, pain, or unprocessed emotions?

Do I have chronic tension in my shoulders, neck, or jaw?

Do I experience stomach issues when I'm anxious?

Do I feel exhausted no matter how much I rest?

Because your body isn't just randomly breaking down.

It's trying to communicate with you.

And if you want to truly heal?

You have to stop treating your body like the enemy—and start working with it instead.

How to Release Stress & Trauma from Your Body

Once I understood that my body was holding onto past stress, trauma, and unresolved emotions, I had to figure out how to release them.

Here's how I started to heal:

1. Understand How Stress & Trauma Affect the Nervous System

Your body has two modes:

1. Fight-or-flight (survival mode)
2. Rest-and-digest (healing mode)

Most people who experience chronic stress, trauma, or long-term illness are stuck in fight-or-flight mode all the time.

This floods the body with cortisol (stress hormones).

It triggers inflammation and worsens pain.

It keeps the immune system on high alert, leading to autoimmune responses.

The key to healing?

Teaching your body that it is safe.

2. Let Go of Stored Trauma Through Movement

Trauma doesn't just exist in your mind.

It lives in your body.

And one of the most powerful ways to release it?

Movements like:

Bouncing on a mini-trampoline – Stimulates the lymphatic system and clears stagnant energy.

Walking in nature – Resets your nervous system and relieves stress.

Yoga & stretching – Releases stored tension in muscles.

Swimming – Soothes the mind and strengthens the body through rhythmic, calming movements.

Because trauma isn't just about what happened.

It's about what got trapped inside you when it did.

And when you move with intention?

You give your body permission to release what it's been holding onto.

3. Use Breathwork to Heal the Nervous System

When you've been living in stress mode for years, your nervous system can get stuck in a constant state of fight-or-flight.

This keeps your body inflamed.

It disrupts your ability to rest and heal.

It keeps your muscles tense and your energy drained.

But breathwork?

It's like a reset button for your nervous system.

One of the simplest breathing techniques I use daily is the 4-7-8 method, introduced by Dr. Andrew Weil, a quick and calming way to reset stress and bring your body back to a place of peace, anytime, anywhere.

The 4-7-8 Breath

1. Inhale deeply through your nose for 4 seconds.
2. Hold your breath for 7 seconds.
3. Exhale slowly through your mouth for 8 seconds.

This instantly signals your body that you are safe, lowering stress and inflammation.

Because when you change your breath?

You change your body's entire response to stress.

4. Prioritize Deep Sleep for Cellular Healing

If there's one thing I've learned, it's this—

Without quality sleep, your body cannot heal.

Sleep is when your body repairs inflammation and damage.

It's when your brain processes and releases emotional stress.

It's when your nervous system fully resets.

Here's what helped me the most:

- Yoga Nidra meditation before bed – Deep relaxation for the nervous system.
- Magnesium supplementation – Helps relax muscles and promote restful sleep.

- A screen-free wind-down routine – Reducing blue light helps improve deep sleep.

Because when you prioritize deep, restorative sleep, your body finally gets the chance to heal from the inside out.

Movement as Medicine: The Nervous System Connection

When I finally began learning about the nervous system, everything fell into place.

My nervous system had been stuck in survival mode for years.

Fight. Flight. Freeze. Fawn.

Always on. Always bracing. Always pushing.

And movement, I realized, could either agitate or regulate it, depending on how I approached it.

When I walked in nature, I felt grounded.

When I stretched slowly, I felt safe.

When I danced to music that made me feel free, I felt alive.

I began to understand this deep truth:

Movement doesn't have to be big to be powerful. It just has to be aligned.

That means moving in ways that don't spike your stress, but soothe your soul.

That means asking your body what she needs—then honoring the answer.

Self-Care Is Not a Luxury—It's Your Lifeline

Movement is just one piece of it.

The other? Rest. Deep rest. Nervous system care. Rituals that bring you home to yourself.

Let me be clear: Rest is not laziness. Rest is repair.

Your body cannot heal when it's constantly under pressure.

And if you're living with chronic illness, burnout, or autoimmune conditions, your nervous system has likely been in overdrive for years.

This is why your self-care cannot wait until you're "less busy."

It cannot be squeezed into the cracks of your day.

It must become your foundation.

This means:

- Prioritizing sleep
- Taking breaks before you crash
- Saying no to overcommitment
- Listening when your body says "not today"
- Practicing gentle movement over punishing workouts
- Creating rituals of stillness, breath, and peace

This is not weakness. This is wisdom.

They Are Learning Too...

The women I coach now are learning what I had to learn the hard way:

- That you don't have to be all or nothing.

- That you don't have to choose between healing and achievement.
- That you don't have to sacrifice your well-being to be worthy.

They are learning to move differently.

To feel again.

To stretch. To walk. To dance. To rest.

To stop seeing their body as a battlefield and start treating it like sacred ground.

They are not waiting to feel perfect before they begin.

They are beginning—imperfectly, intentionally, and with love.

And every time they do, they become more unshakable.

The Breathwork & Meditation Reset

I didn't grow up meditating. In fact, for a long time, the idea felt foreign, like something reserved for yogis or monks, not a woman trying to survive an invisible illness and raise a family. But I reached a point where survival wasn't enough. I wanted to feel peace in my own body. I needed to stop running on fumes and start breathing on purpose.

That's when I found breathwork.

Breath is life. But most of us forget to use it fully. We hold our breath during stress, take shallow inhales, or live in survival mode with tension trapped in our chest. When I began practicing intentional breathwork, I started to feel my nervous system shift. My body softened. My mind slowed down. I wasn't just surviving, I was beginning to heal.

Meditation followed naturally. And no, I didn't sit cross-legged in silence for an hour each day. Some days, it was three minutes of stillness.

Others, it was walking in nature with my eyes open and my heart listening. Meditation isn't about perfection; it's about presence. It's about creating space between the noise of life and the truth inside you.

Whether you call it breath prayer, grounding, or simply taking a sacred pause, it's all part of reclaiming your power. It's part of moving your body with love.

Today, I blend breathwork and meditation into my morning routine. I teach women to reset their energy with one breath, one moment, one decision to slow down and come home to themselves. You don't have to do it perfectly—you just have to begin.

Here's what I want you to remember:

- Your breath is your anchor.
- Stillness is a form of strength.
- Meditation is not escaping life—it's coming back to it.

If no one has told you this before: You're allowed to slow down. You're allowed to breathe. And you're allowed to create space for your own healing.

Blueprint Steps: Move Your Body with Love

1. Ask your body how she wants to move today.

Start each morning with this question. Let your body lead, not your to-do list or guilt.

2. Redefine movement to include softness.

Stretching. Walking. Gentle yoga. Slow dancing. Breathing deeply. It all counts.

3. Protect your rest as much as your movement.

Create sacred rest rituals: establish a consistent bedtime, screen-free nights, and quiet mornings. Guard your energy like it's gold—because it is.

4. Tune into your nervous system.

Notice when you feel calm vs. chaotic. Choose a movement that brings you into regulation, not reactivity.

5. Celebrate what your body can do, without judgment.

Your body is doing her best. Celebrate the steps, not the speed.

- Your body is not a problem to fix. She's a place to come home to.
- Rest is not a reward. It's a requirement.
- You don't have to move harder. You just have to move kinder.
- You are allowed to love your body without needing to change her.
- The body remembers—but she can also release.
- You are allowed to take up space. You are allowed to slow down.
- Every time you move with love, you heal a little more.

6. Breath and Meditate: Reset Your Energy with Stillness

You've celebrated what your body can do. Now honor it with stillness.

Breathwork and meditation aren't luxuries—they're lifelines. They give your nervous system a chance to reset, your mind a chance to soften, and your body the permission to just be.

Even one intentional breath can shift your entire state.

You don't need an hour in silence—just a sacred pause.

Close your eyes. Inhale deeply. Exhale fully. Come home to yourself.

- Your breath is your anchor. Stillness is strength.
- Healing doesn't always come through doing—sometimes, it comes through being.

To You, Beautiful Reader...

You don't have to prove anything.

You don't need to earn your rest or hustle through healing.

You don't need to punish yourself with movement or push through pain just to check a box.

You can move your body from a place of compassion.

From a place of softness.

From a place of enoughness.

Maybe that looks like a five-minute walk.

Maybe it's a stretch on your bedroom floor with candles and quiet music.

Maybe it's dancing in your kitchen with your kids.

Or maybe today, your movement is stillness—and that counts too.

You are allowed to move slowly.

You are allowed to rest.

You are allowed to do what feels good, not what looks impressive.

Because the goal isn't to "get your body back."

The goal is to come home to her.

Journal Prompt: How Do You Want to Feel in Your Body?

Take a few quiet moments to write and reflect:

1. What physical symptoms have you been experiencing lately?
2. What emotions might be connected to those symptoms?
3. What kind of movements make me feel calm, grounded, or joyful?
4. What does your body need from you right now?
5. What's one way I can honor my body this week—with movement or rest?
6. What new story am I ready to write about how I treat and move my body?

Because your body? It keeps the score.

But you have the power to rewrite the story.

_____

_____

_____

_____

_____

_____

_____

_____

Final Words

Healing isn't just about what you eat or how you move.

It's about how you treat yourself—mind, body, and soul.

Unprocessed emotions don't just weigh on your heart. They live in your tissues. It lives in the body. We can stuff it inside ourselves, with nowhere to release it, until we learn that there is a blueprint and a way, emotionally and physically, to listen and honor our body.

And movement, when done with presence, can become the release.

Your body is sacred ground, but so is your spirit.

And the truth is, no amount of movement or mindset work will ever feel fully complete unless you are connected to something deeper.

Because when you've been shaken—physically, emotionally, spiritually— you need more than routines.

You need roots.

That's where we're going next.

In Chapter 7, we'll dive into what it means to connect to faith, purpose, and a calling that carries you, even when everything else feels uncertain.

Because your healing is not just about what you do...

It's about who you are becoming.

Pillar 4 – Connect to Faith and Purpose

It was 3:00 a.m.

The hospital room was cold, sterile, and silent—except for the low hum of machines and the quiet beeping of a monitor beside me.

My body was swollen with inflammation, my joints aching, my heart pounding with fear.

I was alone.

But in that stillness... something stirred.

Tears streamed down my face as I whispered, "God, I can't do this anymore. I'm done fighting. I don't want to live like this. If You're real... I need You now."

I didn't hear a booming voice.

But I felt something I hadn't felt in a long time: peace.

A peace that didn't match my circumstances.

A stillness that wrapped around me like a blanket.

A whisper that rose inside me, saying, "This is not where your story ends."

And right there, in that hospital bed, I knew:

It was time to surrender.

It was time to stop trying to control everything.

It was time to let God in—not just on Sundays or in desperation—but fully, deeply, completely.

That was the moment I awakened—not just physically, but spiritually.

It wasn't just a health crisis.

It was a divine interruption.

And it changed everything.

The Moment I Chose to Let Go and Let God

Until then, I had been doing everything in my own strength.

Pushing through pain. Masking emotions. Carrying the weight of everyone around me. Trying to hold it all together, while I was falling apart inside.

But my body was never the enemy.

It was the messenger.

And the message was clear:

"You were never meant to carry this alone."

That night, I stopped asking "Why me?" and started asking, "What now?"

I asked God for strength.

I asked for clarity.

I asked Him to show me the purpose behind the pain.

And He did.

Not all at once.

Not in a perfectly wrapped moment.

But slowly, gently, over time—through prayer, through stillness, through daily surrender.

My Morning Ritual of Surrender

That awakening didn't end in the hospital.

It began there.

When I returned home, I knew I couldn't go back to life as it was.

I needed daily connection. Daily direction. Daily peace.

So I created a sacred morning ritual.

Nothing elaborate. Just real.

Raw.

Holy.

I'd sit in stillness, and whisper:

"God, I can't do this without You. Please lead me today."

I'd journal what I was grateful for.

I'd read a devotional.

I'd sit in silence long enough to hear my breath—and sometimes, His.

Some days I'd weep.

Some days I'd just sit.

But every morning, I chose to reconnect.

Because the world couldn't wait to pull me into chaos again, but my soul needed calm.

This ritual became my anchor.

My alignment.

My reminder that healing wasn't just about my physical body—it was about my spirit.

Faith Is the Foundation, Not the Last Resort

For so long, I used faith like a fire extinguisher—only grabbing it in emergencies.

But now?

Faith is the foundation of how I live, breathe, heal, and serve.

It's how I start my day.

It's what sustains me when the pain flares.

It's what gives me hope when fear tries to rise.

"Faith is not the absence of struggle."

It's the presence of God in the struggle.

And when you connect to something greater than yourself—when you remember that your life has divine meaning—you stop seeing setbacks as punishments and start seeing them as redirections.

You Are Not Just Here to Survive—You Are Here for a Purpose

If you're reading this right now, feeling broken, overwhelmed, or uncertain, I want to remind you:

You are not an accident.

You are not forgotten.

And you are not disqualified because of your pain.

You are being refined—not rejected.

You are being shaped—not shattered.

You are being rerouted—not ruined.

And the very thing that tried to take you out?

It can become the very thing that lifts others up.

That's what purpose does.

It takes your mess and makes it meaningful.

Journaling, Gratitude & Surrender as a Daily Faith Practice

Each morning, I open my journal and pour it out.

Not just my pain, but my praise.

I write:

- "God, thank You for breath."
- "Thank You for this moment."

- "Even if I don't understand, I trust You."
- "Please guide me today."

And then I write my gratitude.

Some days it's for answered prayers.

Some days it's just, "Thank You for getting me through another night."

And that's enough.

This practice brings me back to faith. Back to trust. Back to the truth.

It reminds me I'm not in this alone.

It reminds me I'm loved, held, and carried—even when I can't see the way forward.

Giving My Pain a Purpose Through Coaching and Storytelling

I didn't set out to become a life coach or a speaker.

But once I started sharing my story—even in small ways—women began saying, "Me too."

"Your words helped me."

"Now I believe I can heal, too."

That's when I realized: My healing wasn't just for me.

It was meant to ripple.

So I leaned in.

I got certified. I built my practice.

I started coaching women who had walked through their own storms—women with autoimmune diseases, anxiety, loss, burnout, pain, overwhelm.

I didn't just coach them.

I saw them.

Because I was them.

And every time I shared a piece of my story—every time I helped someone rewrite theirs—I healed just a little more.

Purpose became my medicine.

Coaching became my calling.

And faith became the fire that fueled it all.

You Can Turn Your Pain Into Purpose Too

You don't have to be a coach or a speaker to serve.

You just have to be willing.

Willing to share what you've walked through.

Willing to sit with someone else in their hard.

Willing to use your voice, your time, your healing, for something bigger.

Because when you stop asking "Why me?" and start asking "Who can I help with this?"

You shift from suffering to service.

And that shift will transform you.

Blueprint Steps: Connect to Faith and Purpose

1. Create a sacred morning ritual.

Start your day with stillness, prayer, or journaling—even if it's just 5 minutes. Let this be your anchor.

2. Surrender daily.

Say this aloud: "God, I release control. Lead me today. I trust You." Then breathe and let go.

3. Write your daily gratitude.

Every morning or evening, write 3 things you're thankful for—no matter how small. Gratitude is faith in motion.

4. Ask how your pain can serve.

What lesson have you learned that someone else might need? Who could your story help?

5. Say yes to your calling.

Whether it's encouraging someone, creating something, or simply showing up with love, your purpose is alive and ready.

- Surrender is not weakness—it's where the strength begins.
- Your story doesn't disqualify you. It qualifies you to help someone else.
- You're not here by accident. You're here on assignment.
- Pain is not the end of the story—it's the opening line of your purpose.
- When you give God your pain, He gives you purpose.
- Your healing isn't just for you—it's meant to ripple.

Journal Prompt: Aligning with Faith and Purpose

1. Where have I been trying to carry it all alone?
2. What does surrender look like for me today?
3. How has my pain shaped me in ways that could serve someone else?
4. What is God inviting me into right now?
5. What would it look like to walk in alignment with faith, peace, and purpose?

Final Words

As your purpose becomes clear, so does your need for protection.

Because when you're walking in your calling, living in alignment, and showing up for others, you must guard your energy and your peace like never before.

That's where we go next.

In chapter 8 of this blueprint, you'll learn how to stop pouring from an empty cup, how to set empowered boundaries, and how to protect the most sacred part of your transformation: your unshakable energy.

Pillar 5 – Protect Your Energy and Set Empowered Boundaries (THE IGNITE Tool™: Your 60-Second Energy Reset)

Have you ever woken up feeling more exhausted than when you went to bed?

As if no matter how much you sleep, drink coffee, or try to push through, your energy is just... gone?

I've been there, too.

And if you've ever whispered to yourself, "Why am I so tired all the time?"—you're not alone.

There was a time in my life when I was constantly running on fumes.

I'd go to sleep tired and wake up feeling even worse.

No amount of coffee helped.

No amount of pushing made it better.

And here's what I finally discovered:

I wasn't just tired. I was energy-depleted.

The Truth About Fatigue That No One Talks About

As someone living with Rheumatoid Arthritis and Fibromyalgia, I know what it's like to be trapped in deep, unexplainable exhaustion.

But what I learned—both as a Registered Nurse and as a woman rebuilding her life—is this:

Fatigue isn't just about sleep.

It's about energy production and protection.

Think of your body like a power plant.

It doesn't just have energy—it creates it through microscopic engines in your cells called mitochondria.

But most of us are treating our bodies like a phone constantly on 1% battery, running all day without ever fully plugging in.

And if you're not fueling that energy or protecting it, your system breaks down.

So What's Actually Zapping Your Energy?

Here's what I learned on my journey back to full-body vitality:

- Lack of deep sleep: Getting less than 6 hours of true rest can reduce your energy production (ATP) by 30%. You're not just tired—you're undercharged.
- Poor hydration: Just a 1% drop in hydration can lead to brain fog, fatigue, and sluggish metabolism. Water is how oxygen gets to your cells. No hydration = no energy.
- Processed food: Sugar and chemicals slow down mitochondrial function. Every bite either fuels your cells or clogs them.

- Stress overload: A single stressful thought can raise cortisol by 23%. Your brain doesn't know the difference between a tiger and a tense email.

So even if you're sleeping eight hours and eating "okay," if you're living in mental overdrive, your energy is leaking faster than you can restore it.

The Turning Point: My Full-Body Breakdown

I was saying yes to too much.

Yes, to people who drained me.

Yes, to obligations I didn't have energy for.

Yes, to proving I could "handle it" even when I couldn't.

But my body was done pretending.

I remember collapsing onto the couch one evening after another long day of ignoring my needs and crying.

Not because something specific happened.

But because I realized I hadn't felt like me in years.

That night, I prayed, "God, I can't live like this anymore. Please show me how to get my energy—and my life—back."

That prayer led me to the kind of transformation that no doctor, no pill, and no amount of caffeine could provide.

Energy Isn't Something You Wait For—It's Something You CREATE

Here's what changed everything:

- I prioritized sleep as if it was my paycheck. Because without rest, healing is impossible.
- I began my mornings in prayer and peace. Not my phone, not my to-do list. Just God, gratitude, and deep breath.
- I moved my body—even just a little. Not to burn calories, but to activate my energy. A five-minute stretch or walk gave me more clarity than any cup of coffee.
- I hydrated like it was medicine because it is.
- I set boundaries like my life depended on it—because it did.

And most of all?

I stopped leaking energy where it wasn't being honored.

Boundaries: The Secret Weapon for Sustained Energy

Boundaries are the bridge back to yourself.

For years, I thought boundaries were walls—something that kept people out or made me less loving, less available, less "nice." I didn't want to disappoint anyone, so I said yes when I meant no. I pushed through exhaustion. I ignored my body's signals. I tolerated too much for too long because I believed love meant sacrifice, and strength meant never saying I needed space.

But I've learned that boundaries are not barriers. They are bridges— back to peace, back to clarity, and back to yourself.

Boundaries are love in action, not just for others, but for you. They're the courageous lines we draw when we finally realize our worth and decide we're no longer available for what drains us, disrespects us, or diminishes us.

It wasn't until I reached a breaking point—mentally, physically, and emotionally—that I saw how vital boundaries were to my healing. My body had been whispering for years: slow down, rest, stop saying yes to everything. But I didn't listen until I had no choice.

And when I finally stopped pushing and started protecting, everything changed.

Boundaries are the blueprint of self-worth

When you set a boundary, you're saying:

"I matter too."

You're reclaiming your voice. You're choosing alignment over obligation. You're giving your nervous system a break from the chaos. You're showing yourself—and others—that your needs are valid and sacred.

At first, it felt uncomfortable. Saying "no" made my heart race. Canceling plans felt selfish. Asking for space triggered guilt. But with time, I realized that every time I honored a boundary, I was rewiring something deep inside. I was healing the belief that I had to sacrifice myself to be loved.

Healthy boundaries are not rejection—they're protection.

They protect your time, values, health, and energy.

They don't push people away—they allow the right people to come close.

Boundaries look like this:

- Saying no without over-explaining
- Letting calls go to voicemail when your soul needs quiet
- Canceling plans when your body says, "Not today"
- Refusing to be pulled into drama or urgency
- Releasing the need to "fix" everyone
- Walking away from one-sided relationships
- Trusting that someone else's disappointment isn't your responsibility to carry
- Giving yourself permission to rest without guilt

It's not always easy. Sometimes you'll be misunderstood. Sometimes others won't like the new version of you who no longer tolerates what once broke you. But that's okay.

You're not here to keep everyone comfortable.

You're here to honor your healing and protect your peace.

Every time you hold a boundary, you teach the world how to treat you, and you remind yourself that your well-being is not up for negotiation.

Setting boundaries is part of living unshakable.

Boundaries allow you to stand firm, even when life gets chaotic. They create space for recovery, clarity, and joy. They give you back the time and energy to focus on what matters most: your health, your family, your purpose, and your light.

This isn't about control. It's about choice.

And boundaries are how you take that choice back.

Boundaries don't make you cold.

They make you clear.

They don't shut people out.

They allow the right people in.

And once I started honoring mine, my whole world shifted.

I protected my mornings. I guarded my peace. I stopped explaining my "no."

And I watched my energy, creativity, and clarity come back online.

Because here's the truth:

You can't pour from an empty cup, and you shouldn't have to.

Movement That Creates Energy

Most people think movement drains you.

But the right kind of movement activates your energy system.

You know who has tons of energy? Kids. Why? Because they move constantly.

As adults, we sit, scroll, worry, and then wonder why we feel dead inside.

You don't need an intense workout. You need a spark.

Try this:

- 5 minutes of jumping jacks or bouncing on a rebounder, mini trampoline.

- A brisk walk outside while breathing deeply.
- A few stretches while listening to calming music.

Movement isn't about exhaustion.

It's about circulation.

It gets the life force moving through you again.

The Invisible Energy Leaks

Let's talk about the real culprits behind your exhaustion.

- Saying yes when you mean no.
- Being "on" for everyone but yourself.
- Mental clutter.
- Toxic conversations.
- Living in fight-or-flight mode 24/7.

Each of these steals your energy, one drop at a time.

And if you don't stop the leaks, no amount of food, sleep, or supplements will fix the fatigue.

You don't need more hustle.

You need more alignment.

To You, Beautiful Reader...

If you feel like you've lost yourself to the demands of life, to exhaustion, to chronic stress—hear this:

You don't need to do more. You need to protect what you already have.

You are allowed to:

- Sleep in.
- Say no.
- Turn off your phone.
- Step back.
- Disappoint people.
- Take up space.
- Honor your body without apology.

You don't need permission to protect your energy.

It was never theirs to take in the first place.

They're Taking Their Power Back Too

The women I coach are learning to say no.

To speak up.

To choose peace over people-pleasing.

To schedule their joy.

To nourish themselves like they matter.

And do you know what happens?

Their minds clear.

Their energy returns.

Their spark ignites.

They stop surviving—and they start thriving.

And you can too.

Your Purest Energy — Protect It

There is a version of you that is vibrant, present, calm, and powerful.

A version that moves from intention, not obligation.

A version that lights up rooms—not because she's trying, but because she's aligned.

That version of you already exists.

But she can't survive in an environment that constantly drains her.

Energy is your most sacred currency.

And while the world will demand more, ask for more, pull for more—you get to decide what you allow.

Protecting your purest energy is a radical act of self-leadership. It's how you preserve your joy, your clarity, and your capacity to serve and live fully.

It took me years to realize this: Not everything deserves access to you.

When you're living with chronic illness, autoimmune conditions, anxiety, or deep emotional wounds, your energy is even more valuable. It takes energy to heal. It takes energy to show up for your family, your dreams, your calling. You don't have time to waste on what isn't life-giving.

So you must become fierce about your peace.

And that begins with awareness.

What drains your energy?

It might be:

- A toxic friendship that always leaves you second-guessing yourself
- Overcommitting your schedule because you're afraid to say no
- Scrolling social media and comparing your journey to someone else's
- Skipping rest because you feel guilty
- Listening to your inner critic instead of your inner truth
- Saying yes out of fear instead of alignment
- Pouring into everyone else and never refilling your own cup

We often feel exhausted, not because we're doing too much, but because we're doing too much that doesn't serve us.

What protects your energy?

- Slowness. Silence. Saying no.
- Time in nature. Breathwork. Stillness.
- Nourishing your body. Listening to music. Laughing with your kids.
- Boundaries. Breaks. Breath.
- Speaking kindly to yourself.
- Releasing the need to explain.
- Being in spaces where you don't have to shrink to fit in.

Protecting your energy is not a one-time decision—it's a daily discipline.

It's choosing again and again to return to yourself.

To let go of what drains and lean into what restores.

This is how you become unshakable.

Not by doing more, but by becoming more intentional.

More selective. More aligned.

You don't owe everyone access to your soul.

You don't have to explain your healing.

You don't need permission to prioritize your peace.

Say this to yourself daily:

"I am worthy of peace. My energy is sacred. I choose to protect what keeps me whole."

Blueprint Steps: Protect and Elevate Your Energy

1. Audit your energy drains.

Write down what's been draining you physically, emotionally, and mentally. Then commit to releasing just one this week.

2. Create a morning peace ritual.

Before checking your phone, take 5 minutes for prayer, silence, or journaling. This sets your nervous system to "safe."

3. Move to activate—not exhaust.

Commit to 5–10 minutes of joyful movement each day: walking, bouncing, stretching, dancing.

4. Hydrate and nourish wisely.

Start each day with lemon water. Eat real food that fuels your cells, not drains them.

5. Set one powerful boundary.

Say no to something that doesn't serve you. Then say yes to something that restores you.

- Energy isn't something you wait for—it's something you create.
- If it costs you your peace, it's too expensive.
- Protecting your energy is a full-time job—and you're the boss.
- You don't have to be available to everyone, all the time, for everything.
- Saying no to them is saying yes to you.
- Rest isn't optional. It's your reset button.
- A peaceful woman is a powerful woman.
- When you elevate your energy, you elevate your entire life.

You've just learned the five core steps I use to protect and elevate my energy every single day. This blueprint changed my life—it gave me the awareness, boundaries, and reset practices I never had when I was stuck in survival mode.

But what about those moments in real time—when you feel overwhelmed, triggered, emotionally off, or completely drained?

Let's be real. You can know what to do and still feel too tired to do it.

That's why I created this.

When I couldn't walk through a full morning routine...

When my nervous system was overloaded and my mind was spiraling...

When I needed something now—not later—I used this reset that I created.

This became my lifeline.

And now, it's yours too.

THE IGNITE Tool™: Your 60-Second Energy Reset

This is your moment-to-moment energy shift. It's how you reset when you feel off, overwhelmed, or emotionally dysregulated. It's not just breathwork—it's a nervous system shift, an intention-setter, and a return to your power in under a minute.

Let's IGNITE:

I – Inhale and Ground

Take a deep inhale. Feel your feet on the floor. Breathe into your belly. Ground yourself back into your body and this present moment.

G – Get Honest

Name what's really going on. "I feel anxious." "I'm overwhelmed." "I'm tired but pretending I'm not." No fixing. Just name it with truth.

N – Name What You Need

Ask: "What do I need right now?" Maybe it's space. Stillness. A walk. A cry. Hydration. Support. Let your nervous system answer, not your to-do list.

I – Interrupt the Pattern

Do one small action to break the energy loop. Step outside. Put your hand on your heart. Say "no" to something. Change your posture. Shift the energy physically.

T – Tap into Gratitude

Name one thing you're grateful for—right here, right now. Gratitude is an instant frequency reset. It shifts you from fear to faith.

E – Exhale and Empower

Release the breath. Let go of what's not yours to carry. Say to yourself, "I choose peace", "I am safe", and "I am powerful." This is your exhale moment of release and re-alignment.

This is your emergency brake and your soul-level reset. Use it when the noise is loud, the stress is high, or your energy feels scattered. It takes just 60 seconds, but it brings you back to yourself—back to your light.

You'll also find this tool in your Unshakable Toolbox at the back of this book for quick access anytime you need it.

"You don't need hours to come home to yourself. You just need a moment of intention, a breath of truth, and the choice to reset. That's how we rise."

Journal Prompt: Elevate and Protect Energy

Take 10 minutes and write from the heart:

1. Where in my life am I leaking energy right now?
2. What am I tolerating that's keeping me tired?
3. What new boundary would feel like self-love to set this week?
4. How can I start each day with peace instead of pressure?
5. What does my highest-energy, most aligned self do differently?

Your Next Level Starts Now

You are not here to stay stuck in survival mode.

You were made for overflow.

And your energy—your light—is the key.

So guard it.

Fuel it.

Move it.

Honor it.

And never again apologize for choosing you.

Because when your energy rises...

Your power follows.

Your healing accelerates.

And your purpose becomes Unshakable.

CHAPTER 9

Pillar 6 – Rise with Resilience (The R.I.S.E. Code™)

There was a time when I felt like my life was slipping away. My body was failing me. The exhaustion was relentless.

I had spent my life as a nurse, a mom, and a strong, capable woman, always taking care of others. But suddenly, I was the one who needed saving. And I had no idea how to rescue myself.

Maybe you've been there. Maybe you're there right now, stuck in a season that feels impossible to get through.

But what if I told you that the very thing trying to break you is actually here to build you? That every challenge, every setback, every moment of doubt is not the end of your story, but the beginning of your comeback?

That's why I developed **The R.I.S.E. Code™**—because resilience isn't just about surviving. It's about rewriting your story, igniting your fire, strengthening your foundation, and elevating into the strongest version of yourself. This is how we rise. This is how we become unshakable.

R – REWRITE YOUR STORY

The greatest battle you will ever fight isn't against your circumstances—it's against the story you tell yourself about them.

For years, I told myself I was broken, that my illness had stolen my future. That I had no control. And the more I believed it, the more I stayed stuck.

But then I asked myself one question that changed EVERYTHING: What if this challenge isn't here to break me, but to build me?

That's when I stopped seeing myself as a victim and started stepping into my power.

I want you to think about the story you've been telling yourself. Have you let your past experiences define you? Have you allowed fear, failure, or setbacks to determine what's possible for your future? Because you don't have to accept the story life hands you. You have the power to rewrite it.

I – IGNITE YOUR FIRE

Resilience isn't about waiting for things to get better. It's about taking action—no matter how small.

When I was at my lowest, I had to make a choice: stay stuck or start shifting. I started fueling my body with healing foods. Moving, even when it was hard. Speaking life over myself instead of fear. And with every small shift, my fire got stronger. Because here's the truth: Your daily choices determine your destiny.

You don't need a massive overhaul to change your life. You need one small shift. One powerful decision. And then another. And another. Until you've built unshakable momentum.

S – STRENGTHEN YOUR FOUNDATION

Breakthroughs don't last without follow-through. This is where most people stop. They start making progress, then life happens, and they slip back into old patterns.

But here's what I teach the women I work with: Resilience isn't built in one big moment. It's built on the quiet, daily commitment to keep showing up.

That's why I use the 1% Rule—just get 1% stronger, 1% braver, 1% better every day. Because small shifts, stacked over time, create unshakable transformation.

The secret to building resilience is acting like the woman you are becoming—**now**—before you feel ready.

E – ELEVATE & EMBODY YOUR NEXT LEVEL

This is where true transformation happens. Because resilience isn't just about rising—it's about stepping fully into the woman you were meant to be.

The strongest version of you is already inside—you just have to elevate into her. Walk like her. Speak like her. Make decisions like her. Embody her strength every single day.

So many of us wait until we "feel" ready to step into our next level. But waiting keeps you stuck. You have to embody that strength now— before you feel confident, before you feel certain, before you have all the answers. The moment you start showing up as your future self, you become her.

Resilience isn't about waiting for life to get easier. It's about becoming stronger. It's about choosing—every single day—to rise, to take up space, and to create a life that isn't defined by your struggles, but by your strength.

Blueprint Steps: The R.I.S.E. Code™

- REWRITE your story: Identify the limiting belief holding you back and replace it with truth.
- IGNITE your fire: Take one small action aligned with your comeback today.
- STRENGTHEN your foundation: Commit to getting 1% better daily—consistency over intensity.
- ELEVATE and EMBODY your next level: Start being her **now,** in mindset, energy, and decisions.

You don't need to be ready. You need to be willing.

Your strength isn't in how little you fall—it's in how often you rise.

Resilience is the bridge between who you were and who you're becoming.

Your next level doesn't wait for your fear to leave. It waits for you to choose.

You don't need to be unstoppable—you just need to be Unshakable.

Journal Prompt: Your Unshakable Comeback

1. What story have I been telling myself, and how can I rewrite it with the truth?

2. What's one small decision I can make today that supports my next-level self?

3. Where do I need to be more consistent and strengthen my foundation?

4. How would the Unshakable version of me think, act, and lead today?

_____

_____

_____

_____

_____

_____

_____

_____

_____

_____

_____

_____

CHAPTER 10

Pillar 7 – Heal Through Love, Forgiveness, and Emotional Freedom

I used to think forgiveness was something I gave to other people. It was a gift I handed to someone who hurt me, whether they deserved it or not. But I've come to realize something far more powerful:

Forgiveness isn't for them. It's for you.

There was a time when I carried so much pain, anger, and disappointment. Pain from my past. From people who didn't show up. From people who said things that cut deep. From situations I didn't ask for and could not change.

But the longer I held on to that pain, the heavier I became. The angrier I got, the more exhausted I felt. And it didn't just affect my mind—it affected my body, my spirit, my energy, and my joy.

I was trying to heal while still holding on to the very things that were keeping me sick.

Forgiveness was the door I needed to open. And love, love was the key.

The Weight We Carry

I want you to imagine carrying a heavy backpack filled with bricks. Each brick represents something or someone you haven't forgiven. Every time you replay that conversation in your head... every time you hold in resentment or bitterness... every time you blame yourself for something in the past... you add another brick.

And then you wonder why you're tired, why you're stuck, why you can't move forward.

Because you can't rise when you're weighed down by pain.

I know what it feels like to be angry at someone who didn't apologize... to blame yourself for things that weren't your fault... to feel ashamed of how long it's taken to heal. But love and freedom don't live in that space.

They live in release.

Forgiveness Is Not Approval, It's Release

Forgiveness doesn't mean you're saying what happened was okay.

It doesn't mean you have to invite that person back into your life.

It means you are done letting that pain take up space inside your soul.

You don't forgive for their benefit.

You forgive to give yourself peace.

Forgiveness is a process, not a one-time event. Some things take time. Some wounds need to be grieved first. But don't let unforgiveness become the thing that holds your healing hostage.

Because you deserve to be free.

The Moment I Learned That Love Is the Most Powerful Healer

There was a time in my life when I believed healing was all about action—the right foods, the right routines, the right strategies.

- I focused on what I needed to change physically—nutrition, movement, and mindset.
- I worked tirelessly to improve my health, thinking I could outwork my pain.
- I held on to resentment toward my body, toward my circumstances, even toward myself.

But I was missing something critical in my healing journey—

The power of love.

Not just love from others, but the deep, transformational power of sending love—intentionally, fully, and without expectation.

It was during some of my hardest moments that I discovered this truth:

Love softens the hardest hearts.

Forgiveness releases the weight we weren't meant to carry.

Kindness—when given freely—creates healing in ways nothing else can.

And when I stopped holding on to resentment and started sending love instead?

Everything changed.

The Truth About Love. Forgiveness & Healing

Most people think love is something that just "happens."

But the truth?

Love is a choice.

A choice to let go of resentment and release past hurts.

A choice to send love even to those who have hurt you, not for them, but for **YOU**.

A choice to lead with kindness, even when it's not easy.

Because holding on to bitterness?

It doesn't protect you.

It poisons you.

But love?

Love sets you free.

You – Where Are You Holding Back Love?

I want you to ask yourself—

Where in your life have you been withholding love?

Is it toward yourself—blaming yourself for things you can't control?

Is it toward someone who hurt you—holding onto pain instead of releasing it?

Is it toward life itself—feeling bitter about your circumstances instead of embracing where you are?

Because here's the truth—

Sending love doesn't mean excusing what happened.

It doesn't mean forgetting.

It means choosing **YOUR** peace over your pain.

And when you do that?

You don't just heal emotionally.

You heal physically, too.

They – How to Send Love & Transform Your Life

Once I realized love was my greatest healer, I made it part of my daily practice.

Here's how you can do the same:

1. Send Love to Yourself First

Most of us are our own worst critics.

We replay past mistakes.

We beat ourselves up over things we can't change.

We hold ourselves to impossible standards.

But the first step to sending love?

Is sending it to yourself.

Here's what I do daily:

- I speak love over myself. (I am worthy, I am enough, I am healing.)
- I release guilt and shame. (I did the best I could with what I knew.)
- I show myself grace. (I deserve kindness—from myself, first.)

Because the more love you give yourself?

The more love you have to give the world.

2. Send Love to Others (Even the Ones Who Hurt You)

This was the hardest for me.

How do you send love to someone who hurt you?

How do you forgive when the pain still feels fresh?

How do you move forward without carrying bitterness?

The answer?

You choose to send love, even when your feelings haven't caught up yet.

It doesn't mean you excuse their actions.

It means you free yourself from carrying it any longer.

One practice that changed my life?

The "Send Love" Visualization

1. Close your eyes and picture the person in front of you.
2. Imagine a soft, warm light surrounding them.
3. Silently say: "I send you love, I release this pain, I choose peace."
4. Breathe deeply and feel the weight lifting.

Because love isn't just about what you give to others.

It's about what you release from yourself.

3. Send Love Into the World Through Kindness

I started asking myself: "How can I show up today with more love?"

- A kind word to a stranger.
- A small act of generosity.
- A moment of presence with someone who needs it.

Because the more love you give, the more love you receive.

And when you make love and kindness your default response?

Your entire life shifts.

The Shift: Leading With Love Changes Everything

I used to think love was soft.

That it was something extra.

That it was secondary to everything else.

But I've learned that love is the strongest force in the world.

It has the power to heal deep wounds.

It has the power to release what's been holding you back.

It has the power to change your life—completely.

And when you make love your foundation?

You become unshakable.

The One in the Mirror

And let's talk about the hardest person to forgive, you.

We are so quick to show grace to others... but brutal with ourselves.

Forgiving myself was the hardest and most necessary part of my healing. I had to forgive myself for not knowing what I didn't know... for how long I stayed stuck... for the way I ignored my needs... for the way I talked to myself when I was hurting.

If you've ever looked in the mirror and only seen flaws, failure, or shame...

If you've ever told yourself, "I should be further along by now..."

If you've ever held a grudge against yourself for past decisions...

It's time to set yourself free.

Because you are not your past. You are not your pain. You are not your mistakes.

You are healing. You are evolving. You are worthy of grace, too.

Healing Through Love and Kindness

After forgiveness, the next step is love.

Not the soft, poetic kind that's only reserved for perfect days or perfect people.

I'm talking about the radical kind of love that meets you in the mess.

The kind of love that says, "Even here, especially here, you are worthy."

When I started showing myself kindness, everything shifted.

I stopped rushing my healing.

I stopped criticizing my progress.

I stopped comparing my journey to anyone else's.

I started treating myself the way I would treat a dear friend, gently, tenderly, with compassion.

And that love? It flowed outward. I began to soften toward others. To understand pain from a place of compassion. To respond instead of react.

Kindness became my medicine.

Love became my fuel.

Forgiveness became my freedom.

Blueprint Steps to Heal Through Forgiveness, Love, and Kindness

1. Acknowledge the wound – be honest about what hurt you and name it.
2. Feel it to free it – allow yourself to grieve and express the emotion. Let the tears come. Healing is not a sign of weakness; it's power.
3. Choose forgiveness – not because they deserve it, but because you deserve peace. Say it aloud, write it, pray it. "I release you. I forgive you. I set myself free.
4. Send love – not to approve of the action, but to release the hold it has over you. Send love and let go.

5. Practice radical kindness – toward yourself and others, as an act of ongoing healing. Do it daily. Speak gently. Rest often. Encourage yourself. Treat yourself with dignity.

6. Speak your release aloud – 'I forgive you, I set myself free.' Even if it takes repeating every day.

Forgiveness doesn't excuse the behavior. It sets you free from being tied to it.

You cannot fully heal while holding onto what hurt you.

Kindness is your superpower—it softens pain, restores connection, and heals hearts.

Forgiveness is how you stop letting the past write your future.

Radical kindness is your reset. Use it often.

The person you most need to forgive might be the one in the mirror.

Love doesn't make you weak. It makes you unshakable.

Journal Prompt: Set Yourself Free

Take 10 minutes and write freely. Let this be your sacred space.

1. What pain or resentment am I still carrying that is weighing me down?
2. Who or what do I need to forgive—not for them, but for me?
3. What would my life feel like if I released that pain today?
4. How can I show radical kindness to myself in this season?
5. What would it look like to send love, even in places where I've been wounded?

CHAPTER 11

Pillar 8 - Lead with Purpose – Share Your Light and Serve from the Heart

I didn't always know this was my purpose. In fact, for a long time, I believed my purpose had passed me by.

I was the woman who showed up for everyone else. I was the nurse, the mom, the wife, the daughter, the friend who always had the answers, the clipboard, the Band-Aid, the prayer. I poured and poured until my cup wasn't just empty, it was shattered.

When illness hit and my world turned upside down, I wasn't thinking about purpose. I was just trying to make it through the day. My body was in pain, my energy was gone, and my confidence felt like it had disappeared with my health. I didn't recognize the woman in the mirror.

But something shifted the moment I realized I didn't have to wait until I was completely healed to begin helping others. That realization changed everything.

Because healing is not the end of the story, it's the beginning of purpose.

You Were Called for More

Maybe you've felt it too, that quiet nudge deep inside that whispers, "You're meant for more."

More than surviving. More than just existing. More than staying small, so others don't feel uncomfortable when you shine.

You're not here by accident. You're here on purpose, with purpose.

Sometimes our greatest purpose is born from the places we once tried to hide. The things we thought disqualified us are, in fact, the very things that equip us to lead. Your story isn't something to be ashamed of—it's your greatest asset. It's your light.

You don't need to be perfect to help others. You just need to be honest. When you lead with heart, people don't need a polished version of you. They need the real you. The one who's been through something. The one who got back up. The one who dared to believe again.

My Shift from Healing to Leading

When I was in the thick of my pain, I didn't know my story would someday be the thing that opened doors, books, platforms, and hearts.

I was journaling to survive. Writing in my gratitude notebook because it was the only thing I could control. I started coaching because I needed something that brought me back to life. I didn't know that the very healing habits I adopted would one day be the blueprint I'd teach to other women.

But I showed up anyway. I shared my story—raw, real, and unfinished.

One by one, women started telling me, "I see myself in your story." And that's when I knew—this was no longer just about me. It was about all of us. I wasn't just reclaiming my health. I was reclaiming my voice. My purpose. My power.

And so are you.

Your Story Carries Light

Your story carries light. Even the chapters you're still healing from. Even the pages you've tried to rip out.

When you give your pain a purpose, it doesn't define you—it empowers you.

Your comeback has meaning. It's not just about what you've been through. It's about what you're going to do with it. Someone needs the wisdom you've earned in the dark.

You don't need a stage to be a light. You can change lives in quiet, sacred spaces. In a conversation over coffee. In a social media post. In the way you show up with empathy and encouragement because you've lived it.

Purpose doesn't require a platform. It only requires a willing heart.

Blueprint Steps: Lead with Purpose and Serve from the Heart

1. Reflect on your healing journey.

Look at what you've overcome—not just what happened, but how you grew. Your story has power because you lived it.

2. Identify the message in your mess.

What would you tell the woman you used to be? What do you wish someone had said to you in your hardest season?

3. Start where you are.

Purpose doesn't wait for perfect timing. You don't need more followers or credentials. Your story is already enough. Your heart is already qualified.

4. Listen to what energizes you.

When you light up while talking about something, pay attention. Purpose and energy are often intertwined. Follow what feels aligned.

5. Be bold enough to speak your story.

Someone is praying for the hope you hold. You never know whose breakthrough will come from your courage to share.

6. Serve with your heart, not your ego.

This isn't about the spotlight. It's about service. Lead with love. Give from overflow, not obligation.

7. Keep showing up.

Purpose isn't a one-time decision. It's a daily devotion. Every act of service, every word of encouragement, every boundary you honor—it's all part of your legacy.

Self-Love: The Soil Where Healing Grows

Healing doesn't happen through pressure, punishment, or perfection.

It happens through love. Gentle, nurturing, consistent love.

You don't need to earn your worth.

You don't need to fix yourself to be lovable.

You don't need to wait until you're "better" to be kind to yourself now.

Self-love is how you come home to yourself.

It's how you soften in the hard moments.

It's how you speak life over your healing.

It's how you rest without guilt and grow without shame.

Self-love is the soil where your Unshakable transformation begins to bloom.

Your Self-Love Declarations

Say these daily. Speak them until they feel real.

- I am enough, exactly as I am.
- I deserve to heal with compassion, not criticism.
- I honor my energy and my needs.
- I release shame and embrace my softness.
- I speak to myself like someone I deeply love.
- I am worthy of love, care, and gentleness—today and always.

Journal Prompt: Return to Love

1. How have I been treating myself lately? Have I been treating myself like someone I love or someone I need to fix?
2. What would it look like to show myself more compassion this week?
3. What is one thing I can do today that nourishes me with love and care?

CHAPTER 12

Pillar 9 – The Power of Tiny Habits that Lead to BIG Change

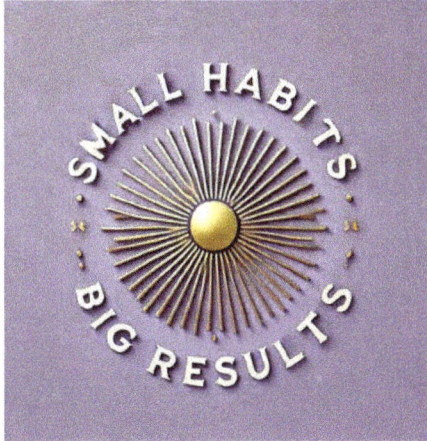

Transformation doesn't happen overnight.

It happens in tiny, consistent decisions—one step, one choice, one moment at a time.

The Myth of the Overnight Fix

For years, I had believed that real change had to be extreme.

I thought if I wasn't doing everything perfectly, it wasn't worth doing at all.

But let me ask you something—

How many times have you set huge goals and then quit when you couldn't maintain them?

How many times have you felt like you were "starting over" because you tried to change too much, too fast?

That's because big, drastic changes rarely last.

Not because we're not capable.

But because our brains and bodies aren't built for sudden, unsustainable shifts.

That's why the key to lasting transformation is starting small.

Not with 10 new habits at once—just one.

Not with perfection—but with progress.

What Small Change Can You Start With?

I want you to think about something.

What is one small change that would move you toward the life you want?

Not five.

Not ten.

Just one.

Because here's the truth—

Your future isn't built by grand gestures.

It's built by the tiny, everyday decisions you make.

- The way you start your morning.
- The thoughts you choose to believe.
- The food you put into your body.
- The way you talk to yourself.

Every single one of these adds up.

So, what's one small change you can commit to—starting today?

The Compound Effect: How Small Choices Create Big Results

When I finally stopped trying to fix everything at once and started focusing on small, consistent actions, my life transformed.

I didn't wake up one morning completely healed.

But I did wake up feeling 1% better.

And that 1% added up—

I started walking outside for 5 minutes every morning. (That turned into 20.)

I swapped my morning coffee for warm lemon water. (That turned into more hydration.)

I started journaling one sentence a day. (That turned into full pages.)

I focused on gratitude for 30 seconds before bed. (That turned into deep, restorative sleep.)

None of these were huge changes.

But together?

They rebuilt my health, my mindset, and my life.

That's the power of the compound effect.

Small, consistent changes lead to massive results.

The Science of Small Wins

There's a reason small changes work better than big ones.

Our brains love quick wins.

Every time you complete a small habit, your brain releases dopamine, the chemical that makes you feel good.

And that feeling?

It builds momentum.

Which means:

The more small wins you get, the more likely you are to keep going.

The easier the new habit feels, the more it becomes part of your identity. The more success you see, the more your confidence grows.

And when your confidence grows?

You start believing in yourself again.

And that belief?

That's when transformation truly begins.

The Rule of 1% Better

If you improve just 1% every day, by the end of the year, you'll be 37 times better than you were when you started.

Not because you did something extreme.

But because you did something small and consistent.

Imagine if you applied this to:

Your health. (One small food swap each day)

Your mindset. (One positive thought replacement each morning)

Your movement. (One extra minute of stretching each night)

Your relationships. (One text to someone you love every day)

1% every day compounds into massive change.

And the best part?

It doesn't feel overwhelming.

Because you're not trying to change everything.

You're just focusing on one small shift at a time.

The Power of Tiny Habits: Where to Start

If you're feeling overwhelmed, here's where you start:

Pick ONE habit. (Not five. Just one.)

Make it ridiculously easy. (So easy it feels impossible to fail.)

Anchor it to something you already do. (Example: Drink water right after brushing your teeth.)

Celebrate the small wins. (Give yourself credit every single time you do it.)

And before you know it?

That small habit becomes part of who you are.

And that's when everything changes.

Because remember: big changes start with one small step.

And that step?

You can take it today.

Journal Prompt: Your 1% Shift

Take a moment to reflect. Grab a journal and answer these questions:

1. What's one small habit that would move you closer to the life you want?
2. What's the easiest way to start implementing it?
3. How can you make it part of your daily routine?
4. How will you celebrate your progress, no matter how small?

CHAPTER 13

Building a Support System: The Importance of Connection

For a long time, the idea of seeking help felt like an admission of failure. My fiercely independent nature, honed over years of battling chronic illness, had instilled a deep-seated belief in self-reliance. Asking for help felt weak, a betrayal of the strength I'd so painstakingly cultivated. I'd built walls around myself, meticulously crafted defenses against vulnerability, convinced that showing weakness would expose me to judgment and further suffering. The truth was, admitting I needed help was terrifying. It meant confronting the limitations of my own resilience, acknowledging the depths of my struggles in a way that felt intensely personal and, frankly, shameful.

This deep-rooted hesitation showed up in subtle ways. I'd minimize my symptoms to friends and family, downplaying the severity of my pain or fatigue. I'd deflect offers of assistance, often with a hastily constructed excuse or a dismissive wave of the hand. I prided myself on my ability to manage my pain on my own, viewing any form of outside support as a potential crutch. The irony, of course, was that this fiercely independent approach was actually hindering my recovery. By refusing to acknowledge my limitations, I was inadvertently prolonging my suffering, creating unnecessary obstacles to healing.

The turning point came gradually, almost unnoticed at first. It started with small concessions, tiny cracks in the walls I'd so diligently constructed. A friend offering to run errands, a family member insisting on bringing over a meal, a colleague offering to cover a shift – these gestures, once met with resistance, started to feel less like a threat and more like a lifeline. I learned that seeking help wasn't a sign of weakness, but a testament to strength. It was a courageous act of self-preservation, a recognition that navigating the complexities of chronic illness didn't have to be a lonely endeavor. Building a support network became a vital part of my healing process, an essential element in my journey towards a fulfilling and meaningful life. The support I received was instrumental in transforming my perspective, shifting my focus from self-reliance to the healing power of connection.

The benefits of accepting help extended far beyond the practical assistance I received. It fostered a deeper sense of connection with myself and others, creating a ripple effect of positive change in my life. The act of receiving support strengthened my self-compassion, allowing me to treat myself with the same kindness and understanding I extended to others. It also deepened my empathy, allowing me to better understand and support those around me who were grappling with their own challenges.

This newfound openness to support extended into my professional life as well. I became more adept at recognizing when I needed help from colleagues and more willing to ask for it. I also became more skilled at recognizing and supporting the needs of my clients, creating a more collaborative and supportive environment for everyone. Building a strong support network isn't just about receiving help; it's about creating a reciprocal relationship, a network of mutual support and understanding.

My journey in seeking and accepting help was a powerful learning experience, a testament to the resilience of the human spirit and the transformative power of connection. It's a lesson I continue to learn and relearn, recognizing that building and maintaining a supportive network is an ongoing process, a commitment to self-care that requires courage, vulnerability, and unwavering self-compassion. It's a journey that has deeply enriched my life, fostering a deeper sense of belonging, resilience, and enduring hope. It's a journey I wholeheartedly recommend to anyone seeking a more fulfilling and meaningful life. The rewards are immeasurable, extending far beyond the practical and touching the very core of our being, shaping our relationships and our understanding of ourselves and the world around us. The power of connection, the strength found in vulnerability – these are the cornerstones of a life lived fully, a life lived with purpose, joy, and unshakable hope.

Finding the right kind of support was crucial, and it didn't happen overnight. It required a conscious effort, a willingness to step outside my comfort zone and embrace vulnerability in a way I'd previously avoided. My initial attempts to connect were tentative, almost hesitant. I dipped my toe into the waters of online support groups, initially lurking in the shadows, reading the posts of others before venturing to contribute my own experiences. The anonymity of the internet provided a certain level of comfort, a buffer against the fear of judgment. I could share my struggles, my fears, and my vulnerabilities without the immediate pressure of face-to-face interaction. Even so, the act of pressing "send" on my first post felt like a leap of faith, a small act of bravery that resonated with a deep sense of vulnerability.

Now that we've built a life of purpose, there's one more thing—

The confidence to own it.

Because living with purpose is one thing.

Owning it unapologetically?

That's where the real transformation happens.

CHAPTER 14

Unshakable Peace: Decrease Stress and Overwhelm

For years, I lived in a constant state of stress, worry, and overwhelm—and I didn't even realize it.

If I'm honest, this was my reality for far too long:

- I was always "on," constantly pushing myself to do more.
- I felt guilty anytime I rested, as if I had to earn my right to slow down.
- My mind was always racing, thinking about what needed to be done next.

I thought this was just how life worked.

I believed I had to keep going, keep pushing, keep proving my worth through action.

But my body?

It was screaming for me to slow down.

At the time, I didn't recognize the toll it was taking, but the signs were there:

- My pain increased.
- My sleep suffered.
- My inflammation flared up.

No matter how well I ate or how much I tried to "manage" my health, the missing piece was clear—

I wasn't managing my stress.

And until I learned how to create true inner peace, nothing else would fully work.

The day I finally gave myself permission to slow down, breathe, and protect my peace—

Everything changed.

And today?

I want to show you how to do the same.

The Truth About Stress & Healing

Most people think stress is just a "mental" issue.

But the truth?

Stress is one of the biggest barriers to healing.

It floods your body with cortisol, increasing inflammation.

It weakens your immune system, making you more vulnerable to illness.

It disrupts your nervous system, keeping you stuck in fight-or-flight mode.

And if you don't actively manage stress?

It becomes your default state.

It drains your energy before the day even starts.

It keeps your body from fully healing, no matter how much else you do right.

This means learning how to manage stress isn't optional.

It's essential.

And once you do?

You unlock a level of clarity, peace, and healing you never knew was possible.

How Is Stress Controlling You?

I want you to ask yourself—

Where is stress showing up in your life?

Are you constantly tense, anxious, or overwhelmed?

Do you struggle to relax, even when you're "resting"?

Does your body feel like it's always on high alert?

Because if stress is running your life, your body is paying the price.

And the good news?

You can take your power back.

The Five Steps to Reducing Stress & Creating Inner Peace

Once I realized stress was blocking my healing, I made it my mission to find ways to release it daily.

Here are the five key strategies that transformed my life and will transform yours, too.

1. Activate Your Body's Relaxation Response

Your nervous system has two modes:

1. Fight-or-flight mode (stress, anxiety, tension).
2. Rest-and-digest mode (calm, healing, relaxation).

Most of us are stuck in fight-or-flight mode all the time.

And the key to healing?

Activating your relaxation response.

One of the fastest ways to do this is through breathwork. When I feel anxiety rising quickly, I use a tool called the physiological sigh shared by Dr. Andrew Huberman, a neuroscientist at Stanford.

What it does: Rapidly reduces stress, lowers cortisol, and calms the nervous system within seconds. It is one of the fastest ways to signal safety to your nervous system.

How to do it:

- Inhale deeply through your nose
- Then take a second short inhale right on top of it(like a double inhale)

Slowly exhale fully through your mouth. Repeat 2-3 times. This tells your nervous system:

"You are safe. You can relax."

And the more you practice this?

The easier it becomes to shift out of stress mode, on demand.

2. Create Boundaries to Protect Your Peace

Most stress doesn't come from what happens to us.

It comes from what we allow:

- Saying yes to things we don't want to do.
- Letting toxic people take up space in our lives.
- Overloading our schedule to the point of exhaustion.

The solution?

Boundaries:

- Say no when something drains your energy.
- Limit time with people who bring negativity.
- Make space for what actually matters.

Because every time you say yes to something that stresses you out?

You're saying no to your peace.

3. Prioritize Sleep for Deep Healing

If there's one thing I've learned, it's this—

Without quality sleep, your body cannot heal.

Sleep is when your body repairs inflammation and damage.

It's when your brain processes and releases emotional stress.

It's when your nervous system fully resets.

But if you're not sleeping deeply?

Your body stays in survival mode.

Your immune system weakens.

Your pain and fatigue increase.

So I started focusing on sleep as a key part of my healing process.

Here's what helped me the most:

- No screens 1 hour before bed – Blue light disrupts melatonin production.
- Yoga Nidra meditation – Deep relaxation to calm the nervous system.
- Magnesium supplementation – Helps relax muscles and promote restful sleep.
- A consistent nighttime routine – Signals the body that it's time to wind down.

Because when you prioritize deep, restorative sleep, your body finally gets the chance to heal from the inside out.

4. Shift Your Mindset from Stress to Peace

One of the biggest breakthroughs in my journey?

Realizing that stress is a choice.

I used to believe I had no control over how I felt.

I thought my circumstances dictated my stress levels.

I blamed outside forces for why I was so overwhelmed.

But then I realized—

Stress doesn't come from what happens to you.

It comes from how you respond.

Now, I actively choose:

Calm over chaos.

Presence over panic.

Peace over pressure.

And every time I do?

I reclaim my energy, my healing, and my power.

The Shift: Becoming Unshakable in Your Peace

Most people chase peace like it's something outside of themselves.

But the truth?

Peace is an inside job.

It's in the way you breathe.

It's in the way you set boundaries.

It's in the way you decide what gets your attention.

And when you choose peace on purpose?

You become unshakable.

No matter what happens around you.

Because your peace?

It's your power.

And it's time to protect it.

Journal Prompt: Releasing Stress & Protecting Your Peace

1. What's the biggest source of stress in your life right now?
2. What's one boundary you can set to protect your energy?
3. How can you start incorporating daily moments of stillness?
4. What does peace feel like in your body, and how can you create more of it?

CHAPTER 15

Living Unshakable—Embracing Strength, Purpose & Inner Peace

Looking back, my transformation is nothing short of miraculous. From a place of constant pain and limitation, I've arrived at a point of vibrant health and purpose. It wasn't a linear path; it was a winding road filled with unexpected twists and turns, setbacks, and moments of intense doubt.

But each challenge, each setback, served as a catalyst for growth, pushing me further toward a life I never thought possible. My days are no longer defined by the relentless cycle of appointments, treatments, and physical limitations. Instead, they are filled with a sense of purpose and joy, a reflection of how resilience and intentional living have changed everything.

My current routine is a far cry from the chaotic existence I once knew. Before my day even begins, I thank God for the gift of being alive- it's something I never take for granted. I name three things I am grateful for before my feet hit the floor, grounding myself in peace and presence. My mornings now begin with freshly made celery juice and a gentle form of movement- whether it's a walk, a few stretches, or time on my mini trampoline. I start the day intentionally, without the noise of my phone, allowing space for calm before anything else. This is followed by a nourishing breakfast, a conscious choice designed to fuel my body and mind with the energy needed to navigate the day. It's not just a routine-it's a lifeline. A peaceful rhythm that fuels my body, steadies my mind, and sets the tone for everything that follows.

The mindful practices I've embraced over the years have strengthened my emotional resilience, helping me face the challenges of healthcare without losing myself to burnout. I've learned to set boundaries, prioritize self-care, and recognize the importance of rest and rejuvenation.

Now, with decades of nursing experience behind me, I'm using my background to help others. I am also enjoying sharing my story as a motivational speaker on resilience and transformation, and living well despite health challenges. I help others see that even in the face of illness, fear, or exhaustion, it's possible to reclaim your life and live well- one choice, one breath, one brave moment at a time.

I find immense fulfillment in my role as a transformational life coach. Helping others navigate their own health journeys, sharing my experiences, and offering guidance has become a powerful source of meaning and purpose. It's a way of giving back, of using my own struggles to empower others.

My coaching sessions are not about offering quick fixes or simplistic solutions; they are about fostering self-awareness, encouraging self-compassion, and empowering individuals to discover their own inner strength and resilience. The connections I've forged with my clients are deeply rewarding, a testament to the power of shared experience and mutual support.

My personal life, too, has undergone a remarkable transformation. Relationships that were once strained by my illness have been strengthened through open communication and shared understanding. Mindfulness has taught me the importance of active listening and empathetic engagement, fostering deeper connections with loved ones. I've learned to cherish the simple moments, the small acts of kindness, the quiet moments of shared laughter and conversation. These are the moments that truly matter, the moments that define the richness of human connection.

My creative pursuits, especially writing, have become a lifeline for expressing my emotions and making sense of everything I've walked through. Writing this book, in particular, has been a deeply meaningful experience– a chance to reflect on the past and understand how far I've come. The act of turning pain into purpose, of shaping my struggles into a story of hope and healing, has brought clarity and peace. It's a reminder of how powerful creativity can be in helping us move forward.

However, my journey is not without its ongoing challenges. There are still days when the physical limitations associated with my chronic illnesses assert themselves. There are moments when fatigue sets in, when pain reminds me of the battles I've fought. But the difference now lies in my ability to respond to these challenges with greater calm and resilience. I no longer view them as insurmountable obstacles, but rather as temporary setbacks offering opportunities for self-compassion and growth.

The mindfulness practices I've cultivated have become an integral part of my life, not just a set of techniques but a way of being. They are woven into the fabric of my daily routine, influencing my interactions, my decision-making, and my overall approach to life. Mindfulness is not about escaping reality; it's about engaging with it fully and authentically, embracing both the joys and the struggles with equal measure.

The key takeaway from my experience is the importance of self-compassion. It's not about self-indulgence or complacency; it's about treating oneself with the same kindness, understanding, and forgiveness that one would offer a cherished friend. It's about acknowledging limitations without self-criticism, recognizing that doing one's best is often enough. Self-compassion is the bedrock of resilience, the foundation upon which a fulfilling life is built.

Through this journey, I've discovered the profound power of gratitude. It's not simply about expressing appreciation for the good things in life but about cultivating a mindset of thankfulness and a recognition of the blessings, both big and small, that enrich our lives. Gratitude fosters a positive outlook, shifts our focus away from what is lacking and toward what we have, and ultimately enhances our sense of well-being.

Moreover, I've learned the importance of setting realistic expectations. The pursuit of perfection is a recipe for disappointment and frustration. Striving for excellence while accepting imperfections is a far more sustainable and rewarding approach. It's about acknowledging the process of growth, embracing the journey, and finding contentment in the present moment.

My journey has been a testament to the fact that chronic illness doesn't have to define a life. It can be a catalyst for profound personal growth, a springboard for creating a life of vibrant health and purpose. Through mindfulness, self-compassion, and an unwavering commitment to self-care, it's possible to navigate the challenges of chronic illness and create a life filled with joy, meaning, and purpose.

My hope is that my story will inspire others facing similar challenges to embrace their own journeys, to discover their inner strength, and to create a life that is not merely about surviving but truly thriving.

The path to thriving is not a destination but a continuous process of growth, learning, and self-discovery. It is a journey of self-acceptance – a journey that requires courage, perseverance, and a deep commitment to oneself. It is a journey worth taking. And it is a journey you can embark on, too.

My Story: From Surviving to Leading Others to Transformation

There was a time when I felt lost in my own struggles—trapped by pain, fear, and the weight of my circumstances.

I was fighting chronic illness.

I was exhausted, physically and emotionally.

I had no roadmap for rebuilding my life.

But when I decided to take back my power, everything changed.

I stopped waiting for circumstances to improve.

I started creating a blueprint for my own healing.

I realized that my journey wasn't just for me—it was meant to help others rise, too.

And that's exactly what I do today.

Coaching, Speaking & My Mission: How I Help Women Step Into Their Power

As a transformational life coach, speaker, and author, I help women:

Break free from limiting beliefs.

Step into their power with confidence.

Create lives filled with strength, peace, and purpose.

Because my mission?

Isn't just about overcoming obstacles.

It's about unlocking the limitless potential within every woman I work with.

The Truth About Transformation

Most people think transformation is:

A destination they'll reach once things are "perfect."

Something reserved for "stronger" or "more capable" people.

Out of reach because they've struggled for too long.

But the truth?

Transformation is available to everyone.

It happens in the small daily decisions, not just the big breakthroughs.

You don't need to wait—you can start creating change TODAY.

That's why I do what I do.

Because I believe in your ability to rise.

And I'm here to guide you through it.

You – Are You Ready to Step Into Your Power?

Ask yourself this:

Are you tired of feeling stuck in the same cycles?

Do you feel like you're meant for more, but don't know how to get there?

Do you want to reclaim your energy, confidence, and purpose?

Then know this:

You don't have to figure it out alone.

How I Help Women Transform Their Lives

Through my work as a coach, speaker, and mentor, I offer women the tools to create lasting transformation.

Here's how I help:

1. Transformational Life Coaching

I work with women who are ready to:

- Break through their fears and step into confidence.
- Shift their mindset from survival mode to thriving.
- Heal from past limitations and create a powerful future.

My coaching programs focus on:

- Mindset mastery – Rewiring negative thought patterns.
- Emotional healing – Releasing stress and past pain.
- Holistic well-being – Strategies to elevate energy and health.
- Actionable steps – Turning vision into reality.

Because coaching isn't about motivation.

It's about transformation.

And when you work with me?

You step into a life you never thought possible.

2. Speaking & Empowerment Events

One of my greatest passions is speaking on stages and leading women through transformation.

I speak on:

- Resilience & Overcoming Limitations – How to rise above challenges and step into strength.
- Healing from the Inside Out – The mind-body connection and how to create true well-being.
- Unlocking Your Potential – How to break through fear and live a purpose-driven life.
- Stress Reduction & Energy Mastery – Practical strategies to restore balance and peace.

I've spoken at summits, and every time I take the stage, my goal is simple:

To ignite something powerful within every woman who hears my words.

Because when you hear a message that speaks to your soul?

You can never go back to who you were before.

3. Writing & Global Impact

Through my book Unshakable and my other published works, I reach women all over the world who:

- Need hope.

- Need a roadmap for healing.
- Need someone who understands what they're going through.

Because my writing isn't just about telling my story.

It's about helping YOU write a new story for your life.

And my mission?

Is to ensure every woman who needs this message gets to hear it.

The Shift: You Are Capable of More Than You Realize

Here's what I want you to know:

You are stronger than you think.

You are more resilient than you realize.

You are capable of creating a life beyond your wildest dreams.

You don't have to stay stuck.

You can rise.

And if you're ready for that transformation?

I'm here to help you make it happen.

Because your journey?

It starts the moment you decide to say yes to yourself.

Journal Prompt: Your Transformation Starts Now

Take a moment to reflect:

1. What's the biggest limiting belief holding you back?
2. What's one small step you can take today to reclaim your power?
3. What would your life look like if you stepped fully into your purpose?
4. How would it feel to finally break free from everything that's been weighing you down?

Next Chapter Preview: Your Unshakable Life Starts Now

Now that we've uncovered how to step into transformation, it's time for the most important piece—

Bringing everything together and making your unshakable life a reality.

In the next chapter, I'll share:

The biggest lessons from this journey.

A powerful call to action for your next steps.

Final words to send you into the world unshakable, fearless, and ready to rise.

Because this book isn't just about reading.

It's about becoming.

And now?

It's your time.

CHAPTER 16

The Journey That Changed Everything – You Are Unshakable

Take a deep breath.

Feel the weight of everything you've learned, every moment of reflection, every realization you've had while reading this book.

You are no longer the same person who started this journey.

Because the woman who first picked up this book?

She was searching for something—hope, answers, a new way forward.

She was tired of feeling stuck in survival mode.

She knew, deep down, that she was made for more.

And now?

She has stepped into her power.

She has ignited her light.

She is transforming her life.

She is unshakable.

Because unshakable isn't something you're born as—it's something you become.

It's in the way you rise when life tries to break you.

It's in the way you choose faith over fear.

It's in the way you refuse to let your past dictate your future.

You are unshakable.

And no one—nothing—can take that from you.

The Truth About Becoming Unshakable

Most people go through life waiting—

Waiting for the perfect moment to start.

Waiting for things to get easier.

Waiting for the fear to disappear before they take action.

But the truth?

There is no perfect moment.

Things don't magically get easier.

Fear doesn't go away—you just learn to move forward anyway.

Being unshakable isn't about never feeling fear.

It's about choosing courage despite it.

It's about showing up for yourself—even on the hard days.

It's about choosing peace over chaos, no matter what's happening around you.

It's about standing tall in the storm—knowing the light inside of you is stronger than anything outside of you.

And the moment you decide that nothing will shake you again?

That's the moment you step into the life you were meant to live.

This is Your Moment

I want you to close your eyes and ask yourself:

What is the life I am meant to live?

What does it feel like to wake up without fear, without limits, without hesitation?

What would change if I stopped waiting and started stepping into my power now?

How would my life look if I truly believed that I am unshakable?

Because here's the truth—

You were never meant to stay small.

You were never meant to live in fear.

You were never meant to just survive—you were made to thrive.

And now?

It's time to rise.

How to Live Unshakable Every Day

The greatest lesson I've learned in my journey.

Being unshakable isn't a one-time decision.

It's a choice you make every single day.

And if you want to live this truth every day, here's how:

1. Own Your Story—Every Part of It

For years, I let my struggles define me.

I saw my illness as a limitation.

I saw my setbacks as proof that I wasn't strong enough.

I carried my past pain like a weight I could never put down.

But here's what I've learned—

Your past does not define you.

Your challenges are not your identity.

Every struggle you've faced has prepared you for your breakthrough.

The moment you own your story—every broken piece, every hard chapter, every battle you've fought—

That's the moment you reclaim your power.

Because your story?

It's not a tragedy.

It's your testimony.

And the world needs to hear it.

2. Protect Your Peace Like Your Life Depends On It (Because It Does)

Most of us are exhausted not because we do too much, but because we carry too much.

We carry other people's opinions.

We carry stress that isn't ours to bear.

We carry guilt for taking care of ourselves.

But the key to living unshakable?

Protecting your peace like it's the most valuable thing you own.

If it drains you? Let it go.

If it doesn't align with your purpose? Say no.

If it steals your joy? Walk away.

Because your energy? It's sacred.

And the more you protect it, the stronger you become.

3. Ignite Your Light & Transform Your Life

You were born with a light inside of you—one that cannot be dimmed, no matter how much darkness you've faced.

But if you want to transform your life?

You have to ignite that light and let it shine.

Be bold enough to take up space.

Be fearless enough to show up as your true self.

Be unshakable enough to keep going—even when it's hard.

Because the world doesn't need you to shrink.

It needs you to rise.

4. Walk in Your Purpose & Never Look Back

I used to wonder—

"What if I fail?"

"What if I'm not good enough?"

"What if I try and nothing changes?"

But then I asked myself—

"What if I'm meant for more than I ever imagined?"

And that?

That's when everything changed.

Because when you walk in your purpose:

Doors open that you never expected.

Opportunities flow toward you instead of you chasing them.

You become magnetic to everything meant for you.

And when you commit to never looking back?

You create a future more powerful than you ever dreamed possible.

The Shift: You Are Made for More

I need you to hear this:

You are powerful.

You are capable.

You are made for more.

No matter what you've been through.

No matter what you thought was impossible.

No matter how long you've been stuck.

You can rise.

You can transform.

You can live a life that is truly unshakable.

Because the only thing standing between you and the life you were meant to live?

Is the moment you decide to claim it.

And that moment?

Is now.

Final Journal Reflection: Step Into Your Power

This book was never just about my story.

It's about yours, too.

And now?

It's time to write your next chapter.

Make it unshakable.

1. What does being unshakable mean to me?
2. How am I committing to living unshakable every day?
3. What's the first action I will take to step fully into my power?

Final Words

Pat yourself on the back; you've almost reached the end of this book.

But this?

It's just the beginning of your transformation.

You are no longer the woman who started this journey.

You are stronger.

You are bolder.

You are unshakable.

Now go live like it.

Ignite your light.

Transform your life.

Never doubt that you are made for more.

And when the world tries to shake you?

Stand tall and shine brighter.

Because you, my friend?

Are Unshakable.

Becoming Unshakable

There comes a moment in every woman's life when she realizes she can't go back—not to who she was, not to who the world told her to be. She has walked through too much fire, cried too many silent tears, and survived too many storms. But instead of breaking her, those moments built her.

I know, because I lived it.

I didn't write this book from the mountaintop. I wrote it from the valley—the hospital bed, the sleepless nights, the moments I felt like giving up. And I wrote it from the rise—the moment I chose to believe that I could still heal, still rise, still shine. That's what being unshakable means.

It doesn't mean life won't shake you. It means you remember who you are when it does.

This is What It Means to Be Unshakable

Being unshakable is not about pretending to be strong. It's about choosing to stand in your truth, even when your knees tremble. It's about rising again and again with love for yourself, grace for your journey, and fire in your soul.

Throughout this book, we've walked together through the blueprint that changed my life:

- Fueling your body with love, not punishment

- Mastering your mindset and rewriting your inner dialogue
- Moving your body with compassion
- Reconnecting with your faith and purpose
- Protecting your energy and honoring your boundaries through **The IGNITE Tool™**
- Turning setbacks into comebacks through **The R.I.S.E. Code™**
- Forgiving yourself and others to heal through love and kindness
- Leading with purpose and serving from the heart

This isn't just a blueprint. It's a way of being. A new identity. A declaration that you are more than your pain, your past, or your diagnosis. You are light. You are power. You are Unshakable.

You Don't Have to Be Fully Healed to Rise

Let go of the idea that you need to be "ready" to begin. You are already becoming. Healing is not linear. It's not a checklist. It's a remembering. A returning. A reclaiming of everything that life tried to take from you.

You are not here to shrink. You are here to shine.

You are not broken. You are becoming.

You are not weak. You are rising.

Even when it's messy. Even when you fall. Even when it's hard to believe. You are still rising.

That's the difference between surviving and transforming. That's the difference between fear and fire.

That's the unshakable life.

To the Woman Reading This

I wrote this book for the woman who wakes up exhausted before the day begins.

For the woman who doesn't recognize herself in the mirror anymore.

For the woman who wonders if she's too far gone to come back.

Let me tell you something from the deepest place in my soul:

You are not too far gone. You are right on time.

You are allowed to take your power back.

You are allowed to love yourself in your lowest moments.

You are allowed to rest, to breathe, to rise slowly, and still be worthy of everything good.

You are allowed to walk away from what drains you and run toward what heals you.

And most of all, you are allowed to be both healing and powerful at the same time.

Let This Book Be Your Beginning

Let it be the moment you chose something different.

Let it be the reason you started showing up for yourself again.

Let it be the catalyst that reminds you that you were never defined by your diagnosis, your past, or anyone else's opinion.

Let it be the spark that woke up your light.

Because you were never meant to live dimmed, and you were never meant to stay buried in shame, fear, or fatigue.

You were made to rise. You were made to lead. You were made to live fully, despite your limitations, and especially because of them.

Your pain isn't your prison. It's your platform.

Your breakdown isn't your end. It's your beginning.

Your comeback? It starts now.

What Comes Next

Take the blueprint. Make it your own. Let it guide you as you rise into the version of yourself you were always meant to be.

Let it remind you that healing is not a linear process, and strength doesn't mean perfection.

If you're ready to go deeper, to rise faster, to be held and supported in your transformation, I would be honored to walk with you.

Visit www.sonyamcdonald.com to learn more about my coaching, speaking, and upcoming events.

You don't have to do this alone. You were never meant to.

Moments to Remember

- You don't need to be fully healed to be fully powerful
- Your pain isn't your identity—it's your teacher
- You are allowed to be a masterpiece and a work in progress
- Your worth was never in question
- You are not here to survive—you are here to shine

- The most powerful version of you? She's already inside
- Healing isn't about becoming someone new; it's remembering who you were before the world forgot your light.

Final Words: Rise Now

This is not the end. This is the beginning.

Now you rise.

You rise with light.

You rise with purpose.

You rise with love.

You rise with fire.

You rise Unshakable.

And the world won't be the same because of it.

With all my heart,

Sonya

The Unshakable Toolbox – Tools That Transform

These are the healing tools, habits, and mindset practices that helped me shift from surviving to living well despite limitations. I didn't find them in a textbook—I lived them. These tools helped me rise from pain, fear, and burnout into purpose, peace, and clarity.

I'm not sharing them to overwhelm you. I'm sharing them because even one of these can change everything. Start small. Stay consistent. And trust that every shift counts.

Mindset & Emotional Reset Tools

- **The R.I.S.E. Code™** – A transformational blueprint for building resilience, reclaiming identity, and elevating energy with an unshakable mindset.

  REWRITE your story: Identify the limiting belief holding you back and replace it with truth.

  IGNITE your fire: Take one small action aligned with your comeback today.

  STRENGTHEN your foundation: Commit to getting 1% better daily—consistency over intensity.

  ELEVATE and **EMBODY** your next level: Start being her **now**, in mindset, energy, and decisions.

- **Daily Gratitude Journaling** – Ground yourself in what's working, even in the storm.
- **Visualization** – If you can see it in your mind, you can move toward it.
- **Rewriting Your Story** – You are not your past. You can choose a new narrative.
- **Affirmations** – Speak life over yourself. Every. Single. Day.
- **Meditation** – Create stillness to reconnect with your body and truth.

Nervous System & Energy Tools

- **The IGNITE Tool™** – A 60-second reset to shift energy fast through intention and breath.

This is your moment-to-moment energy shift. It's how you reset when you feel off, overwhelmed, or emotionally dysregulated. It's not just breathwork—it's a nervous system shift, an intention-setter, and a return to your power in under a minute.

Let's IGNITE:

I – Inhale and Ground

Take a deep inhale. Feel your feet on the floor. Breathe into your belly. Ground yourself back into your body and this present moment.

G – Get Honest

Name what's really going on. "I feel anxious." "I'm overwhelmed." "I'm tired but pretending I'm not." No fixing. Just name it with truth.

N – Name What You Need

Ask: "What do I need right now?" Maybe it's space. Stillness. A walk. A cry. Hydration. Support. Let your nervous system answer, not your to-do list.

I – Interrupt the Pattern

Do one small action to break the energy loop. Step outside. Put your hand on your heart. Say "no" to something. Change your posture. Shift the energy physically.

T – Tap into Gratitude

Name one thing you're grateful for—right here, right now. Gratitude is an instant frequency reset. It shifts you from fear to faith.

E – Exhale and Empower

Release the breath. Let go of what's not yours to carry. Say to yourself, "I choose peace." "I am safe." "I am powerful." This is your exhale moment of release and re-alignment.

- **Breathwork** – A powerful way to release stress and ground yourself in the present.
- **Walking in Nature** – Nature has a frequency that calms, restores, and recharges.
- **Ocean Swims or Cold Rinses** – Shock the system gently. Refresh. Reset.
- **Yoga Nidra** – A form of deep rest that restores both the body and the brain.

Body & Nourishment Tools

- **Celery Juice & Anti-Inflammatory Foods** – Your food is your fuel. Heal from within.
- **Gentle, Compassionate Movement** – Listen to your body. Move with love, not punishment.
- **Sleep Rituals** – Wind down with intention. Protect your rest like your life depends on it—because it does.
- **Hydration & Supportive Supplements** – Small, simple choices that support your healing daily.

Faith & Soul Practices

- **Prayer** – My anchor, my compass, my conversation with God.
- **Sunrises & Sunsets** – Symbolic reminders that every day is a new beginning.
- **Forgiveness Work** – Releasing pain to make room for peace.
- **Serving Others with Purpose** – Turning your pain into purpose brings deep healing.

Daily Affirmations to Live an Unshakable Life

Speak Life Over Yourself

Here's a beautiful and powerful collection of affirmations focused on worthiness and being enough. Speak these over yourself daily, especially on the days you forget how powerful, worthy, and loved you are.

I am enough, exactly as I am.

I don't have to earn my worth—it was mine all along.

Even on my hardest days, I am still worthy of love and kindness.

I am allowed to take up space, to rest, and to be seen.

I don't need to do more to deserve more. I already am more.

My value is not tied to what I achieve, but to who I am.

I am not behind. I am right on time for my own journey.

Being kind to myself is not selfish—it's sacred.

I release the belief that I have to be perfect to be worthy.

I am worthy of peace, even when life feels chaotic.

I speak to myself with gentleness, compassion, and grace.

I am not a problem to fix—I am a person to love.

I honor all parts of me—the healing, the hurting, the growing.

I am safe to be seen, safe to rest, and safe to be real.

I let go of the voice that says I'm not enough.

I am deeply loved by God, just as I am.

I am not broken—I am becoming.

I am enough even when I feel undone.

My worth is not up for debate.

I show up for myself with the same love I give to others.

I am learning to love myself out loud.

I choose to see myself through the lens of love, not lack.

I am deserving of tenderness, even from myself.

I forgive myself for the times I forgot my worth.

I am worthy of joy, healing, and beautiful new beginnings.

I am not defined by my diagnosis.

I am healing—body, mind, and soul.

I choose to honor my body with love, grace, and compassion.

My limitations do not limit my worth.

I can live well, even in the midst of challenges.

I am stronger than I feel and braver than I know.

I release the need for perfection and embrace progress.

Every day, I choose peace over pressure.

I trust my body's wisdom and listen with love.

My story is not over. I am still becoming.

I let go of what no longer serves me and welcome what uplifts me.

I am allowed to rest without guilt.

Healing is not linear, and I honor my journey.

I am more than my pain—I am purpose in motion.

I wake up each day with hope in my heart and light in my soul.

I create space for joy, even in the small moments.

I am whole, even while healing.

I give myself permission to thrive, not just survive.

I am worthy of a beautiful life, no matter what I've been through.

I choose faith over fear and love over lack.

I am Unshakable.

Unshakable Daily Affirmations

There is power in the words you speak—especially the ones you say to yourself.

Use this page daily. Read them aloud. Write them in your journal. Post them on your mirror. Let these truths become part of your healing, your hope, and your becoming.

I am worthy of love, healing, and joy.

I am enough, just as I am today.

I honor my body, my story, and my strength.

I choose to speak to myself with kindness and grace.

I am allowed to rest without guilt.

I am safe to be real, soft, strong, and human.

I trust the timing of my healing journey.

I release the need to prove my worth, because it's already mine.

I am more than my limitations.

I choose faith over fear and self-love over self-criticism.

My story is still unfolding—and it's a powerful one.

I give myself permission to be both a masterpiece and a work in progress.

I forgive myself for the days I forget how far I've come.

I choose to see myself through a lens of love and compassion.

Every day, I am becoming more aligned with who I truly am.

I am not behind—I am blooming on time.

I radiate light, purpose, and unshakable strength.

I am loved by God, held in grace, and guided by purpose.

I deserve a beautiful life, no matter what I've walked through.

Today, I choose peace. Today, I choose myself.

In your healing journey, your mindset is everything. Speaking life, love, and truth over yourself each day is not just a practice—it's a declaration. These affirmations are here to anchor you when fear rises, when doubt creeps in, or when the old story tries to pull you back.

You can also include a Journal Prompt right after:

1. Which affirmation do I most need today?
2. Why does this truth matter to me right now?
3. How can I embody it in my words, choices, and mindset today?

Which of these affirmations speaks to your soul right now? Write it down, speak it!

YOU ARE UNSHAKABLE – A Poem written by Sonya McDonald

You've walked through storms and danced through pain,
Turned every loss into radiant gain.
You've shattered doubt, reclaimed your voice,
You rise each day—you own your choice.

You're not defined by past or fear,
Your light burns bold, forever clear.
You shine so bright, you won't be dimmed,
Your power flows from deep within.

You're not your labels, not your scars,
You're made of light, you reach for stars.
You've broken chains that used to bind—
You rise unshaken, soul aligned.

You are unshakable—watch you ignite,
Transform your life and blaze with light.
No fear can hold, no weight can break—
You were born to rise, not to break.

So if you've fallen, hear this line:
Your truth, your fire, was made to shine.
You're not your pain, you're not your past—
You are unshakable. Built to last.

Read this when you forget who you are. Then rise and shine.

About the Author

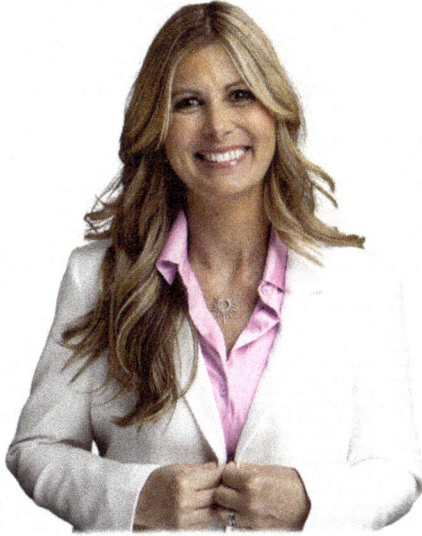

Sonya McDonald is a Keynote Speaker, National and International Bestselling Author, Board-Certified Transformational Life Coach trained by the Robbins-Madanes Institute, Registered Nurse, and Certified Breathwork and Meditation Facilitator. With over 30 years of experience as a Registered Nurse, Sonya blends her medical expertise with holistic healing, mindset transformation, and energy restoration to help others rise above fear, burnout, and invisible illness.

She is the creator of **The Energy Intelligence Method™**, a 9-pillar blueprint designed to help women reduce inflammation, reclaim energy, and live well, despite limitations.

Diagnosed in her 30s with Rheumatoid Arthritis and Fibromyalgia, Sonya knows the pain of losing your identity to illness. After years of exhaustion, prescriptions, and fear, a hospitalization in 2020 became her awakening. She made a decision to stop merely surviving and start living intentionally, with grace, compassion, and clarity.

Her transformation began with a deep shift: honoring her body, reconnecting to faith, and building a life around healing. She incorporated daily practices like celery juice, anti-inflammatory nutrition, journaling, visualization, breathwork, meditation, and yoga nidra—tools that now form the core of her healing system and blueprint.

Sonya's work bridges the gap between science and soul. She helps women regulate their nervous systems, release internalized stress, and rewrite their stories through powerful daily practices. Her signature **IGNITE Tool™: a 60-Second Energy Reset** grounded in breath, intention, and energy redirection, has helped clients around the world move from burnout to clarity. She also created **The R.I.S.E. Code™— her transformational blueprint for building resilience, reclaiming identity, and elevating energy with an unshakable mindset.**

Her debut solo book, **Unshakable: Unlocking Your Blueprint to Living Well Despite Limitations**, is a raw, powerful journey through darkness, healing, and awakening. In it, she shares her step-by-step blueprint for transformation, guiding readers to reconnect with their bodies, shift their energy, and embrace the truth that healing is possible, no matter what they face.

Sonya's story has been featured on NBC News and will soon be seen on Recipe for Wellness Season 2 on PBS, as well as in multiple bestselling anthologies. She speaks on national stages, leads transformational retreats, and coaches women who are ready to live fully and fiercely, without apology.

Her message is clear:

You are not your diagnosis. You are not broken. You are powerful, capable, and made for more.

When she's not coaching or speaking, Sonya finds peace walking her dog at sunrise, soaking in ocean swims, and watching sunsets by the beach. She treasures time with her husband and two beautiful daughters, and lives each day grounded in gratitude, anchored in faith, and fueled by the belief that healing is possible for everyone.

Her signature message:

Ignite Your Light. Transform Your Life. Live an Unshakable Life.

To book Sonya for your next event or schedule a free Energy Health Assessment, visit www.sonyamcdonald.com

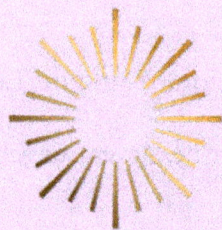

"The power to transform
your life begins with
a single step: choosing
to believe in your own light"

- Sonya McDonald

Connect With Sonya

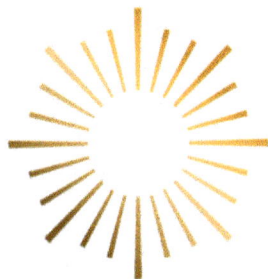

Sonya McDonald

Transformational Life Coach, RN, BSN, BCC

Ignite Your Light. Transform Your Life. Live an Unshakable Life.

Website: https://www.sonyamcdonald.com

LinkedIn: https://www.linkedin.com/in/sonya-mcdonald-rn-bsn-bcc-7786521b9/

Facebook: https://www.facebook.com/sonya.mcdonald.96

Instagram: https://www.instagram.com/sonyamcdonald_/

YouTube: https://www.youtube.com/@sonyamcdonald11